Athletic Training and Performance

Athletic Training and Performance

Edited by
Tom Donnelly

Larsen & Keller
www.larsen-keller.com

Athletic Training and Performance
Edited by Tom Donnelly
ISBN: 978-1-63549-724-3 (Hardback)

Larsen & Keller
Published by Larsen and Keller Education,
5 Penn Plaza,
19th Floor,
New York, NY 10001, USA

Cataloging-in-Publication Data

Athletic training and performance / edited by Tom Donnelly.
p. cm.
Includes bibliographical references and index.
ISBN 978-1-63549-724-3
1. Physical education and training. 2. Athletic ability. 3. Sports medicine.
I. Donnelly, Tom
GV206 .A85 2018
796--dc23

The publisher's policy is to use permanent paper from mills that operate a sustainable forestry policy. Furthermore, the publisher ensures that the text paper and cover boards used have met acceptable environmental accreditation standards.

Printed and bound in China.

For more information regarding Larsen and Keller Education and its products, please visit the publisher's website www.larsen-keller.com

Table of Contents

Preface

As an allied healthcare profession, athletic training refers to the practice and study of providing best professional care to athletes. It includes diagnosis, prevention and treatment of injuries and acute and chronic diseases. Athletic training has five major domains - therapeutic intervention, injury and illness prevention, examination and diagnosis, healthcare administration and immediate care. This book is compiled in such a manner, that it will provide in-depth knowledge about the theory and practice of athletic training and performance. It attempts to understand the multiple branches that fall under this field. This textbook attempts to assist those with a goal of delving into the field of athletic training and performance.

Given below is the chapter wise description of the book:

Chapter 1- Athletic training is the training received by trainers and health care professionals. It consists of the diagnosis and prevention of injuries that can cause any type of disability to the athlete. This chapter will provide an integrated understanding of athletic training.

Chapter 2- Endurance training is the training undergone by athletes to increase their strength. Endurance training can be divided into two categories, general and specific. Strength training, cross-training and physical exercise are some of the exercises discussed in the following section. The major components of athletic training and performance are discussed in this chapter.

Chapter 3- There are various injuries faced by athletes during their athletic activities. Catastrophic injury, shin splints, tennis elbow, golfer's elbow and anterior cruciate ligament injury are some of the injuries faced by athletes. Athletic training and performance can best be understood in confluence with the major topics listed in the following chapter.

Chapter 4- The branch of medicine which deals with injuries caused by physical exercise is known as sports medicine. The common types of injuries that occur because of sports are muscle cramps, ACL tears, shin splints, concussion, muscle strains and ACL sprains. This chapter discusses sports medicince in a critical manner providing key analysis to the subject matter.

Indeed, my job was extremely crucial and challenging as I had to ensure that every chapter is informative and structured in a student-friendly manner. I am thankful for the support provided by my family and colleagues during the completion of this book.

Editor

1

A Brief Introduction to Athletic Training

Athletic training is the training received by trainers and health care professionals. It consists of the diagnosis and prevention of injuries that can cause any type of disability to the athlete. This chapter will provide an integrated understanding of athletic training.

Athletic Training

Athletic training has been recognized by the American Medical Association (AMA) as an allied health care profession since June 1991.

"Athletic training is practiced by athletic trainers, health care professionals who collaborate with physicians to optimize activity and participation of patients and clients. Athletic training encompasses the prevention, diagnosis, and intervention of emergency, acute and chronic medical conditions involving impairment, functional limitations and disabilities."

There are five domains of athletic training listed in the 7th edition (2015) of the Athletic Training Practice Analysis:

- Injury and Illness Prevention and Wellness Promotion
- Examination, Assessment and Diagnosis
- Immediate and Emergency Care
- Therapeutic Intervention
- Healthcare Administration and Professional Responsibility

An athletic trainer functions as an integral member of the health care team in clinics, secondary schools, colleges and universities, professional sports programs, and other athletic health care settings.

History

Athletic training in the United States began in October 1881 when Harvard University hired James Robinson to work conditioning their football team. At the time, the term "athletic trainer" meant one who worked with track and field athletes. Robinson had worked with track and field athletes and the name "athletic trainer" transferred to those working on conditioning these football players and later other athletes. Athletic trainers began to treat and rehabilitate injuries in order to keep the athletes participating. The first major text on athletic training and the care of athletic injuries was called Athletic Training (later changed to The Trainer's Bible) written in 1917 by Samuel E. Bilik. Early athletic trainers had "no technical knowledge, their athletic training techniques usually consisted of a rub, the application of some type of counterirritant, and occasionally the prescription of various home remedies and poultices". In 1918, Chuck Cramer started the Cramer Chemical Company (now Cramer Products) that produced a line of products used by athletic trainers and began publishing a newsletter in 1932 entitled The First Aider.

An organization named the National Athletic Trainers' Association (NATA) was founded in 1938 and folded in 1944. Another NATA was founded in 1950 and still exists. The first athletic training curriculum approved by NATA was in 1959 and the amount of athletic training programs began to grow throughout colleges and universities in the United States. In the early development of the major, athletic training was geared more towards prepping the student for teaching at the secondary level, emphasizing on health and physical education. This program was first introduced at an undergraduate level in 1969 to the schools of Mankato State University, Indiana State University, Lamar University, and the University of New Mexico.

Through the years athletic training has evolved to be defined as "health care professionals who specialize in preventing, recognizing, managing, and rehabilitating injures". During the 1970s the NATA Professional Education Committee formed a list of objectives to define athletic training as a major course of study and to eliminate it as a secondary-level teaching credential. By June 1982, there were nine NATA-approved graduate athletic training education programs. On July 1, 1986, this work was used to implement athletic training as a major course of study in at least 10 colleges and universities, and to only start the development of the major in a handful of others.

Once athletic training was recognized as an allied health profession the process of accrediting programs began. NATA's Professional Education Committee (PEC) was the first to take on this role of approving athletic training educational programs. The AMA's Committee on Allied Health Education and Accreditation (CAHEA) was given the responsibility in 1993 to develop requirements for the programs of entry-level athletic trainers. At this time all programs had to go through the CAHEA accreditation process. A year later CAHEA was broken up and replaced with the Commission on Accreditation of Allied Health Education Programs (CAAHEP), which then lead the accreditation process. In 2003 JRC-AT, Joint Review Committee on Athletic Training completely took over the process and became an independent accrediting agency like all other allied health professions had. Three years later JRC-AT officially became the Committee for Accreditation of Athletic Training Education (CAATE), which is fully in charge of accrediting athletic training programs in the United States. NATA produced the NATABOC in 1969 in order to implement a certification process for the profession for an entry-level athletic trainer. In 1989, became an independent non-profit corporation and soon later changed its name to the Board of Certification (BOC).

Roles and Responsibilities

Scope

The Board of Certification serves as the national certifying body for athletic trainers, and its Standards of Professional Practice outline the roles and responsibilities of certified athletic trainers. Such practice standards include practice expectations such as, "The Athletic Trainer renders service or treatment under the direction of a physician." Regardless of the setting, limitations and restrictions on what an athletic trainer can do and who can be treated are in large part determined by the regulatory statutes governing professional practice in individual states.

Referring

"In certain situations, an individual may require treatment from or consultation with a variety of both medical and nonmedical services and personnel other than the athletic trainer." It is the athletic trainer's responsibility to understand the limits of their scope of practice and recognize situations where a referral is necessary. "A number of support health services may be used including school health services, nurses, physicians, dentists, podiatrists, physician's assistants, physical therapists, strength and conditioning specialists, biomechanists, exercise physiologists, nutritionists, psychologists, massage therapists, occupational therapists, emergency medical technicians, paramedics, chiropractors, orthopedists, prosthesis, equipment personnel, referees, or social workers."

NATA Code of Ethics

"The National Athletic Trainers' Association Code of Ethics states the principles of ethical behavior that should be followed in the practice of athletic training. It is intended to establish and maintain high standards and professionalism for the athletic training profession."

Employment Settings

- Clinic
- Hospital
- Industrial/Occupational
- Corporate

- College/University
- Two-year Institution
- Secondary School
- Professional Sports
- Amateur/recreation/youth sports
- Performing Arts
- Military/Law Enforcement/Government
- Health/fitness/sports/performance enhancement clinics/clubs
- Independent Contractor

Education

Undergraduate Course Descriptions

All courses may have prerequisites to be completed before taking further coursework. Also, those prerequisites and content of the courses will vary upon the institute and professor. The courses listed below are commonly taken to increase knowledge regarding athletic training.

- Human Physiology- This course is designed to provide students with an understanding of the function and regulation of the human body and physiological integration of the organ systems to maintain homeostasis.
- Human Anatomy- The anatomical structures of the body will be studied in this course. Including the muscular systems, organs, respiratory, bony anatomy, veins and arteries. This course will help you to learn all components of the body and is almost always accompanied with a lab section to reinforce the lectures.
- Exercise Physiology- This course investigates the acute responses and chronic adaptations of physiological functions to a wide range of physical exercise conditions, involving people of all ages and abilities.
- Kinesiology- Structural and applied musculoskeletal anatomy relative to human movement and sports skill. This course concentrates on muscles, their origins, insertions, and actions.
- Nutrition- This course emphasizes basic nutritional principles and concepts, their application to personal health and relationship between food and its use by the human body for energy, regulation, structure, and optimal health. Discussion of issues in nutrition during various stages of the life cycle and specific chronic diseases will be addressed.

- Therapeutic Modalities- This is a course looks into the background for clinical application of therapeutic modalities in athletic training. Students will comprehend the underlying theories, physiological effects, indications, and contraindications of various therapeutic modalities utilized in the treatment of orthopedic injuries.
- Acute Care of Injury and Illness- This course focuses on the emergency management techniques that are commonly implemented when dealing with trauma and illnesses suffered during/through sport participation. Included will be field evaluation of medical emergencies, such as cessation of breathing or circulation, shock, concussion, and spinal injury to the athlete. Students will review policies and position statements issued by the NATA, NCAA, ACSM, AAP, and AMA regarding prevention, evaluation, and management of acute athletic injuries and illnesses.
- Physical Examination of the Lower Extremities- Intense in-depth study of the lower extremities including physical examinations, injury recognition, treatment, taping, bracing, and care. Laboratory experiences emphasize the methods and techniques in evaluating lower extremity injuries/conditions.

Undergraduate Athletic Training Programs

The Commission on Accreditation of Athletic Training Education (CAATE) website provides a list of all the accredited programs in the United States. It provides you with the name of the college, who to contact, and a link to the institution's website. An Undergraduate Athletic Training degree can only be received at an accredited school for athletic training.

Entry-level Masters Programs

Although the majority of athletic trainers receive a bachelor's degree in athletic training before taking the Board of Certification Exam (BOC), it is not the only way to receive an education in athletic training. An entry-level masters program is a two-year program that covers the same material as an undergraduate athletic training degree. Common prerequisite classes are human anatomy, human physiology, kinesiology, biomechanics, exercise physiology, nutrition, and personal health along with a certain number of observation hours completed under the supervision of a certified athletic trainer (ATC). Prerequisites can vary by institution so be sure to research the prerequisites for your institutions of interest. There are 26 accredited entry level masters programs in the U.S.A.

Graduate School in Athletic Training and Related Fields

There are approximately 15 accredited athletic training masters programs. These programs consist of students who are already certified athletic trainers that want to advance their academic and clinical experience. These are two-year programs which culminate with a Master of Science degree (M.S.) in athletic training. Graduate programs in athletic training are not always specifically in athletic training, but in a related field. Some of these fields may include, but are not limited to, kinesiology, biomechanics, sports management, sport and exercise psychology, exercise physiology, health promotion, etc. These programs are also two years in length. While enrolled in one of these programs, the athletic trainer may gain clinical experience and receive a stipend through a make some money by obtaining a graduate assistantship.

Graduate Assistant Position

A graduate assistant athletic trainer position is a position in which a graduate athletic training student is able to work as an assistant athletic trainer while taking graduate courses. Graduate assistant athletic trainers are responsible for providing the medical coverage of select teams at the institution where they are working. Responsibilities may vary, but include administering daily medical coverage for selected intercollegiate athletic teams (practice/event); traveling with the assigned team, evaluation and documentation of athletic injuries, administrative responsibilities, serve as Approved Clinical Instructor (ACI) or Clinical Instructor (CI) in a CAATE – accredited ATEP, and other duties as assigned by the head athletic trainer. Other responsibilities may include working at a high school, clinic, teaching, or doing research. Graduate assistant positions are generally about 10-month appointments that are renewable after the first year, and may include additional summer work. Visit the National Athletic Trainers' Association Career Center for job postings.

Accredited Programs

Athletic Training programs are evaluated by CAATE to ensure that they follow the standards for Entry-Level Athletic Training Programs. Evaluations may take place every three to seven years depending on the results of the last visit. Successfully completing the CAATE accredited education program is a part of the criteria that determines a candidate's eligibility for the Board of Certification (BOC) examination.

Organizations

"The National Athletic Trainers' Association (NATA) is the professional membership association for certified athletic trainers and others who support the athletic training profession. Founded in 1950, the NATA has grown to more than 35,000 members worldwide today. The majority of certified athletic trainers choose to be members of the NATA – to support their profession, and to receive a broad array of membership benefits. By joining forces as a group, NATA members can accomplish more for the athletic training profession than they can individually".

Before the formation of NATA, athletic trainers occupied a somewhat insecure place in the athletic program. Since that time, as a direct result of the standards and ethics established by NATA, there has been considerable professional advancement. Every year

NATA works on behalf of all athletic trainers to enhance health care for both athletic trainers and those who receive care.

NATA is the professional organization for Athletic trainers across the nation. Each region of the USA has their own district under NATA but within their area, they have their own agendas and board members. Each district also has a director that serves on the NATA Board of Directors.

Every state has their own state athletic training association that acts similar to the district associations as they have their own board members. The state associations answer to the district associations and the National Athletic Trainers' Association. Links to the state associations can be found through the regional websites.

Current Topics

Due to the physicality of athletics and the campaign for healthy well-being, there are issues that become hot topics in the media. Athletic trainers have to continually be aware of changes in laws, position statements of the National Athletic Trainers Association, and institutional policies.

Current hot topics and topics to keep an eye on include:

- NATA Press Room
- Concussion laws, position statements, and policies.
- Youth Sports Legislation
- Guidelines in Prevention of Chronic Overuse Injury in Pediatric Patients
- Athletic Trainers as Physician Extenders
- Education on Public Safety in the Workplace
- Certified Athletic Trainer as a partner in the Athletic Department

Athletics (Physical Culture)

Athletics is a term encompassing the human competitive sports and games requiring physical skill, and the systems of training that prepare athletes for competition performance. Athletic sports or contests, are competitions which are primarily based on human, physical competition, demanding the qualities of stamina, fitness, and skill. Athletic sports form the bulk of popular sporting activities, with other major forms including motorsports, precision sports, extreme sports and animal sports.

Athletic contests, as one of the earliest types of sport, are prehistoric and comprised a significant part of the Ancient Olympic Games, along with equestrian events. The word "athletic" is derived from the Ancient Greek word (athlos) meaning "contest". Athletic sports became organized in the late 19th century with the formation of organizations such as the Amateur Athletic Union in the United States and the Union des Sociétés Françaises de Sports Athlétiques in France. The Intercollegiate Athletic Association of the United States (later the NCAA) was established in 1906 to oversee athletic sports at college-level in the United States, known as college athletics.

Athletics has gained significant importance at educational institutions: talented athletes may gain entry into higher education through athletic scholarships and represent their institution in an athletic conference. Since the Industrial Revolution, people in the developed world have adopted an increasingly sedentary lifestyle and as a result athletics now plays a significant part in providing routine physical exercise. Athletic clubs worldwide offer athletic training facilities for multitudes of sports and games.

Etymology

The word athletics is derived from the Greek word "athlos", meaning "contest" or "task." The Ancient Olympic Games were born of war and featured various forms of athletics such as running, jumping, boxing and wrestling competitions.

In the modern English language, the term athletics has taken on two distinct meanings. Its meaning in American English connotes human physical sports and their respective systems of training. The other principal meaning of the word comes from British English and variants within the British Commonwealth; this meaning of athletics refers solely to the concept of the sport of athletics (a category of sporting competition which comprises track and field sports and various forms of foot racing), rather than athletic activity in general.

Biological Factors

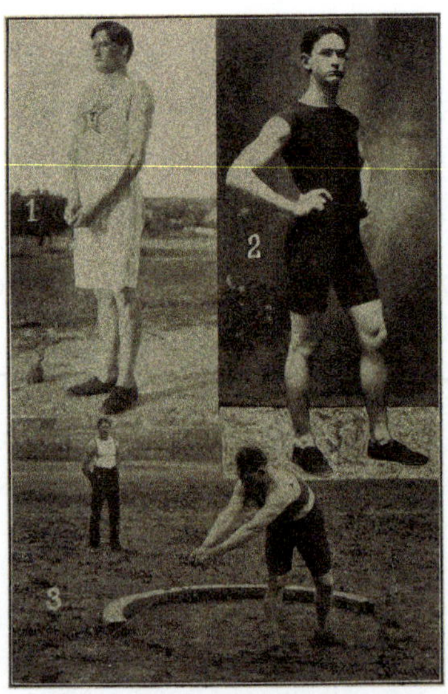

A few athletes

Sex and genetics play major roles in athletic body types. There are significantly fewer football leagues for women; however, women have been active in martial arts for centuries, and sports like figure skating and tennis tend to favor women in terms of spectator popularity. Basketball, high jump, and volleyball favor taller athletes, while gymnastics and wrestling favor shorter ones. Long distance runners tend to be thinner, while competitive powerlifters and American football players tend to be stockier. Athletic development often begins with athletic parents.

Physical conditioning is a primary athletic function for competition. Most often, trainers utilize proven athletic principles to develop athletic qualities; these qualities include coordination, flexibility, precision, power, speed, endurance, balance, awareness efficiency, and timing. While physical strength is prized over most other qualities in Western athletics, it is forbidden in the physical conditioning of T'ai chi ch'uan.

Sports medicine not only treats injuries with medical procedure, but attempts to prevent problems such as trauma and overuse injuries. Sports medicine can also include the use of massage, glucose testing, Rolfing, physical therapy, and performance-enhancing drugs like caffeine and anabolic steroids.

Sports nutrition is the study and practice of nutrition and diet as it relates to athletic performance. It is concerned with the type and quantity of fluid and food taken by an athlete, and deals with nutrients such as vitamins, minerals, supplements and organic substances such as carbohydrates, proteins and fats. Although an important part of many sports training regimens, it is most intensely applied in strength sports (such as weight lifting and bodybuilding) and endurance sports (for example cycling, running, swimming).

Training and Coaching

Athletes first learn basic movement patterns such as running, stopping, jumping and throwing. Coaches help athletes refine these movements into sport specific skills. A skill such as high jumping can then be refined into a competitive technique like the Western roll or the Fosbury Flop. An individual's expression of a technique is often called a style; while various competitive swimming strokes are also called styles. Team sports often develop and practice plays or strategies where players carry out specific tasks to coordinate a team effort of attack or defense.

Technical training may also include teaching the rules and restrictions of a sport or game.

Elite athletes and teams require high-level coaching. A coach is often associated only with an athlete's technical development; however, a coach will likely play all the roles of mentor, physical trainer, therapist, medical responder, technical trainer and performance facilitator. Coaches may or may not involve sportsmanship in their program. Coaching typically signifies a quadrennial, ongoing mentorship for athletic development, as opposed to a clinician who might only assist for a short period of time.

Not only must coaches be able to teach technical form, but recognize and correct problems with a teams' or an athlete's technique and conditioning. Recent advancements in video technology can provide accurate biomechanical data to optimize the form, precision, timing, efficiency and power of an athlete's movements.

Critical to a team's or an athlete's success is a winning attitude. Inherent in the drive to win is the ability to remain relaxed and focused under the pressure of competition. Modern athletic coaches employ the use of sports psychologists to help athletes organize themselves through visualization, relaxation techniques, self-talk, concentration, etc.

Amateurs and Professionals

Title IX of the Education Amendments of 1972 was created to prohibit sex discrimination in education programs that receive (U.S.) federal funding. The original statute made no reference to athletics or athletics programs. From 1972 to 2006, Title IX underwent a series of amendments for gender equity which became high impact on high school and collegiate athletics because it promoted maximum female participation in athletics through equal spending.

Professional sports are sports in which athletes receive payment for their performance. Professional athletics is seen by some as a contradiction of the central ethos of sport, competition performed for its own sake and pure enjoyment, rather than as a means of earning a living.

Organizations

- International Olympic Committee
- National Collegiate Athletic Association
- Amateur Athletic Union
- Union des Sociétés Françaises de Sports Athlétiques
- International Association of Athletics Federations
- Chin Woo Athletic Association
- National Association of Intercollegiate Athletics
- Association for Intercollegiate Athletics for Women

Athletic Trainer

An athletic trainer is a certified and licensed health care professional who practices in the field of sports medicine. Athletic training has been recognized by the American Medical Association (AMA) as an allied health care profession since 1990.

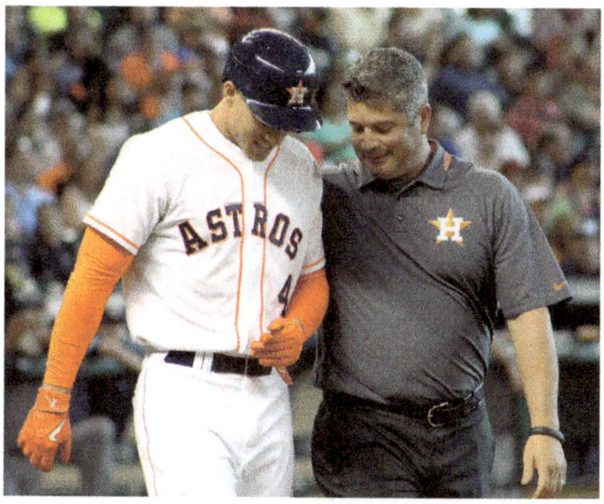

Athletic trainer Nate Lucero (*right*) evaluates Houston Astros baseball player George Springer after Springer was hit by a pitch in 2014

As defined by the Strategic Implementation Team of the National Athletic Trainers' Association (NATA) in August 2007:

"Athletic training is practiced by athletic trainers, health care professionals who collaborate with physicians to optimize activity and quality of life for patients both of the physically active and sedentary population. Athletic training encompasses the prevention, diagnosis and intervention of emergency, acute and chronic medical conditions involving impairment, functional limitations and disabilities."

To become an athletic trainer one must have a master's degree from an accredited professional level education program and then sit for and pass the Board of Certification (BOC) examination. Each state then has their own regulatory agencies that control the practice of athletic training in their state. Most states (42) require an athletic trainer to obtain a license in order to practice in that state, 5 states (Colorado, Hawaii, Minnesota, Oregon, West Virginia) require registration, 2 states (New York, South Carolina) require certification, while California has no state regulations on the practice of athletic training. Areas of expertise of certified athletic trainers include:

- Apply protective or injury-preventive devices such as tape, bandages, and braces
- Recognize and evaluate injuries
- Provide first aid or emergency care
- Develop and carry out rehabilitation programs for injured athletes
- Plan and implement comprehensive programs to prevent injury and illness among athletes
- Perform administrative tasks such as keeping records and writing reports on injuries and treatment programs

Services rendered by the athletic trainer take place in a wide variety of settings and venues, including actual athletic training facilities, primary schools, universities, inpatient and outpatient physical rehabilitation clinics, hospitals, physician offices, community centers, workplaces, and even the military. Emerging settings for athletic training include surgical fellowship opportunities.

Educational Programs

The Commission on Accreditation of Athletic Training Education (CAATE) oversees the curriculum standards of all accredited Professional (entry level) and all of the institutions. The standards dictate the content of both didactic and clinical practice portions of the educational program. Content areas include:

- Risk Management and Injury Prevention
- Pathology of Injuries and Illnesses
- Orthopedic Clinical Examination and Assessment
- Medical Conditions and Disabilities
- Acute Care of Injuries and Illnesses
- Therapeutic Modalities
- Conditioning and Rehabilitative Exercises
- Psychosocial Intervention and Referral
- Nutritional Aspects of Injuries and Illnesses
- Healthcare Administration
- Professional Development and Responsibility
- Healthcare Professional Development and Responsibility

Post-professional Programs

There are several post-professional master's-level athletic training programs. These programs are for credentialed athletic trainers who desire to become scholars, researchers, and advanced practice professionals. Schools with post-professional athletic training masters programs include: A.T. Still University, University of Hawaii at Manoa, Illinois State University, Indiana State University, Indiana University, University of Kentucky, Michigan State University, Western Michigan University, University of North Carolina Chapel Hill, Ohio University, University of Oregon, California University of Pennsylvania, Temple University, Old Dominion University, University of Toledo, University of Virginia, University of Missouri, Weber State University, University of Michigan.

There are doctoral programs in athletic training, each with different curricular emphasis. Athletic training program in doctoral education is offered by the University of Idaho, A.T. Still University, and Indiana State University.

Treatment Population and Settings

Athletic trainers treat a broad population, from the amateur and professional athlete to the typical patient in need of orthopaedic rehabilitative care. The NATA describes typical clients groups as:

- Recreational, amateur and professional athletes
- Individuals who have suffered musculoskeletal injuries
- Those seeking strength, conditioning, fitness and performance enhancement
- Others designated by the physician.

Services rendered by the athletic trainer take place in a wide variety of settings and venues. These may include:

- Athletic training clinics
- Schools (K-12, colleges, universities)
- Outpatient Rehabilitation Clinics
- Hospitals
- Physician offices
- Community facilities
- Workplaces (commercial and government)
- Military installations and veteran medical facilities
- Professional sport organizations

Sport of Athletics

Athletics or track and field is a collection of sporting events that involve competitive running, jumping, throwing, and walking. The most common types of athletics competitions are track and field, road running, cross country running, and race walking.

The results of racing events are decided by finishing position (or time, where measured), while the jumps and throws are won by the athlete that achieves the highest or furthest measurement from a series of attempts. The simplicity of the competitions, and the lack of a need for expensive equipment, makes athletics one of the most commonly competed sports in the world. Athletics is mostly an individual sport, with the exception of relay races and competitions which combine athletes' performances for a team score, such as cross country.

Organized athletics are traced back to the Ancient Olympic Games from 776 BCE. The rules and format of the modern events in athletics were defined in Western Europe and North America in the 19th and early 20th century, and were then spread to other parts of the world. Most modern top level meetings are conducted by the International Association of Athletics Federations and its member federations.

The athletics meeting forms the backbone of the Summer Olympics. The foremost international athletics meeting is the IAAF World Championships in Athletics, which incorporates track and field, marathon running and race walking. Other top level competitions in athletics include the IAAF World Cross Country Championships and the IAAF World Half Marathon Championships. Athletes with a physical disability compete at the Summer Paralympics and the IPC Athletics World Championships.

Initially, the term was used to describe athletic contests in general – i.e. sporting competition based primarily on human physical feats. In the 19th century, the term athletics acquired a more narrow definition in Europe and came to describe sports involving competitive running, walking, jumping and throwing. This definition continues to be the most prominent one in the United Kingdom and most of the areas of the former British Empire. Furthermore, foreign words in many German and Roman languages which are related to the term athletics also have a similar meaning.

In much of North America, *athletics* is synonymous with sports in general, maintaining a more historic usage of the term. The word "athletics" is rarely used to refer to the sport of athletics in this region. *Track and field* is preferred, and is used in the United States and Canada to refer to most athletics events, including racewalking and marathon running (although cross country running is typically considered as a separate sport).

History

Antiquity

Athletic contests in running, walking, jumping and throwing are among the oldest of all sports and their roots are prehistoric. Athletics events were depicted in the Ancient Egyptian tombs in Saqqara, with illustrations of running at the Heb Sed festival and high jumping appearing in tombs from as early as of 2250 BC. The Tailteann Games were an ancient Celtic festival in Ireland, founded around 1800 BCE, and the thirty-day meeting included running and stone-throwing among its sporting events. The original and only event at the first Olympics in 776 BCE was a stadium-length running event known as the *stadion*. This later expanded to include throwing and jumping events within the ancient pentathlon. Athletics competitions also took place at other Panhellenic Games, which were founded later around 500 BCE.

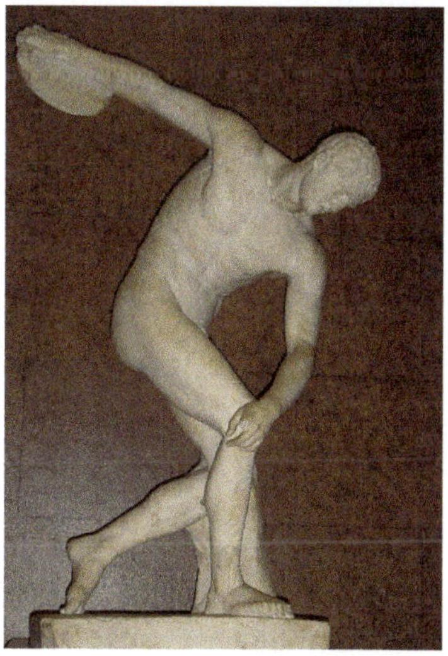

A copy of the Ancient Greek statue *Discobolus*, portraying a discus thrower

Modern Era

The Cotswold Olimpick Games, a sports festival which emerged in 17th century England, featured athletics in the form of sledgehammer throwing contests. Annually, from 1796 to 1798, L'Olympiade de la République was held in revolutionary France, and is an early forerunner to the modern summer Olympic Games. The premier event of this competition was a running event, but various ancient Greek disciplines were also on display. The 1796 Olympiade marked the introduction of the metric system into the sport.

Athletics competitions were held about 1812 at the Royal Military College, Sandhurst, and in 1840 in Shrewsbury, Shropshire at the Royal Shrewsbury School Hunt. The Royal Military Academy at Woolwich held an organised competition in 1849, and a regular series of closed meetings open only to undergraduates, was held by Exeter College, Oxford from 1850. The annual Wenlock Olympian Games, first held in 1850 in Wenlock, England, incorporated athletics events into its sports programme.

The first modern-style indoor athletics meetings were recorded shortly after in the 1860s, including a meet at Ashburnham Hall in London which featured four running events and a triple jump competition.

The Amateur Athletic Association (AAA) was established in England in 1880 as the first national body for the sport of athletics and began holding its own annual athletics competition – the AAA Championships. The United States also began holding an annual national competition – the USA Outdoor Track and Field Championships – first held in 1876 by the New York Athletic Club. Athletics became codified and standardized via the English AAA and other general sports organisations in the late 19th century, such as the Amateur Athletic Union (founded in the US in 1888) and the Union des sociétés françaises de sports athlétiques (founded in France in 1889).

An athletics competition was included in the first modern Olympic Games in 1896 and it has been as one of the foremost competitions at the quadrennial multi-sport event ever since. Originally for men only, the 1928 Olympics saw the introduction of women's events in the athletics programme. Athletics is part of the Paralympic Games since the inaugural Games in 1960. Athletics has a very high-profile during major championships, especially the Olympics, but otherwise is less popular.

An international governing body, the International Amateur Athletics Federation (IAAF), was founded in 1912; it adopted its current name, the International Association of Athletics Federations, in 2001. The IAAF established separate outdoor World Championships in 1983. In modern times, athletes can receive money for racing, putting an end to the so-called "amateurism" that existed before.

The Comité International Sports des Sourds had been formed by 1922, to govern international deaf sports, including athletics.

The first organized international competitions for athletes with a physical disability (not deaf) began in 1952, when the first international Stoke Mandeville Games were organized for World War II veterans. This only included athletes in a wheelchair. This inspired the first Paralympic Games, held in 1960. Competitions would over time be expanded to include mainly athletes with amputations, cerebral palsy and visual impairment, in addition to wheelchair events.

Events

The International Association of Athletics Federations, the sport's governing body, defines athletics in five disciplines: track and field, road running, race walking, cross country running, and mountain running. All forms of athletics are individual sports with the exception of relay races. However, athletes' performances are often tallied together by country at international championships, and in the case of cross country the finishing positions of the top athletes from each team or country are combined to declare a team victor.

Track and Field

Track and field competitions emerged in the late 19th century and were typically contested between athletes who were representing rival educational institutions, military organisations and sports clubs. Participating athletes may compete in one or more events, according to their specialities. Men and women compete separately. Track and field comes in both indoor and outdoor formats, with most indoor competitions occurring in winter, while outdoor events are mostly held in summer. The sport is defined by the venue in which the competitions are held – the track and field stadium.

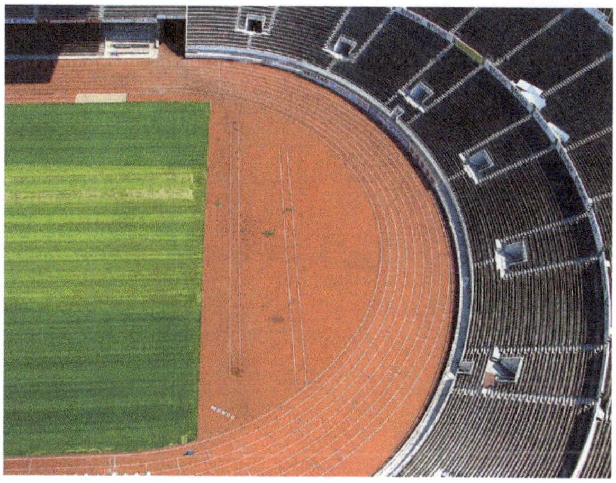

A typical track and field stadium with an oval running track and a grassy inner field

A variety of running events are held on the track which fall into three broad distance categories: sprints, middle-distance, and long-distance track events. Relay races feature teams comprising four runners each, who must pass a baton to their team-mate after a specified distance with the aim of being the first team to finish. Hurdling events and the steeplechase are a variation upon the flat running theme in that athletes must clear obstacles on the track during the race. The field events come in two types – jumping and throwing competitions. In throwing events, athletes are measured by how far they hurl an implement, with the common events being the shot put, discus, javelin, and hammer throw. There are four common jumping events: the long jump and triple jump are contests measuring the horizontal distance an athlete can jump, while the high jump and pole vault are decided on the height achieved. Combined events, which include the decathlon (typically competed by men) and heptathlon (typically competed by women), are competitions where athletes compete in a number of different track and field events, with each performance going toward a final points tally.

The most prestigious track and field contests occur within athletics championships and athletics programmes at multi-sport events. The Olympic athletics competition and World Championships in Athletics, and the Paralympic athletics competition and IPC World Championships in Athletics, are the highest and most prestigious levels of competition in track and field. Track and field events have become the most prominent part of major athletics championships and many famous athletes within the sport of athletics come from this discipline. Discrete track and field competitions are found at national championships-level and also at annual, invitational track and field meets. Meetings range from elite competitions – such as those in the IAAF Diamond League series – to basic all comers track meets, inter-sports club meetings and schools events, which form the grassroots of track and field.

Official world championship track and field events								
Track					Field		Combined events	
Sprints	Middle-distance	Long-distance	Hurdles	Relays	Jumps	Throws		
60 m 100 m 200 m 400 m	800 m 1500 m *3000 m*	5000 m 10,000 m	*60 m hurdles* 100 m hurdles 110 m hurdles 400 m hurdles 3000 m steeplechase	4×100 m relay 4×400 m relay	Long jump Triple jump High jump Pole vault	Shot put Discus throw Hammer throw Javelin throw	*Pentathlon* Heptathlon Decathlon	

Road Running

Road running competitions are running events (predominantly long distance) which are mainly conducted on courses of paved or tarmac roads, although major events often finish on the track of a main stadium. In addition to being a common recreational sport, the elite level of the sport – particularly marathon races – are one of the most popular aspects of athletics. Road racing events can be of virtually any distance, but the most common and well known are the marathon, half marathon, 10 km and 5 km. The marathon is the only road running event featured at the IAAF World Championships in Athletics and the Summer Olympics, although there is also an annual IAAF World Half Marathon Championships. The marathon is also the only road running event featured at the IPC Athletics World Championships and the Summer Paralympics. The World Marathon Majors series includes the five most prestigious marathon competitions at the elite level – the Berlin, Boston, Chicago, London, and New York City marathons.

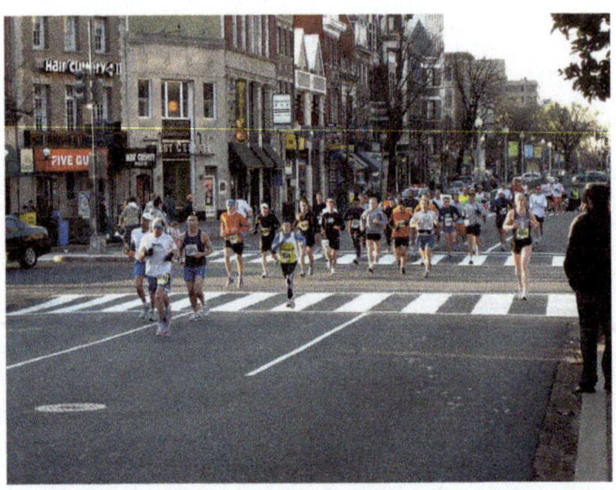

Runners in the popular National Marathon race in Washington, D.C

The sport of road running finds its roots in the activities of footmen: male servants who ran alongside the carriages of aristocrats around the 18th century, and who also ran errands over distances for their masters. Foot racing competitions evolved from wagers between aristocrats, who pitted their footman against that of another aristocrat in order to determine a winner. The sport became professionalised as footmen were hired specifically on their athletic ability and began to devote their lives to training for the gambling events. The amateur sports movement in the late 19th century marginalised competitions based on the professional, gambling model. The 1896 Summer Olympics saw the birth of the modern marathon and the event led to the growth of road running competitions through annual events such as the Boston Marathon (first held in 1897) and the Lake Biwa Marathon and Fukuoka Marathons, which were established in the 1940s. The 1970s running boom in the United States made road running a common pastime and also increased its popularity at the elite level.

Ekiden contests – which originated in Japan and remain very popular there – are a relay race variation on the marathon, being in contrast to the typically individual sport of road running.

Cross Country Running

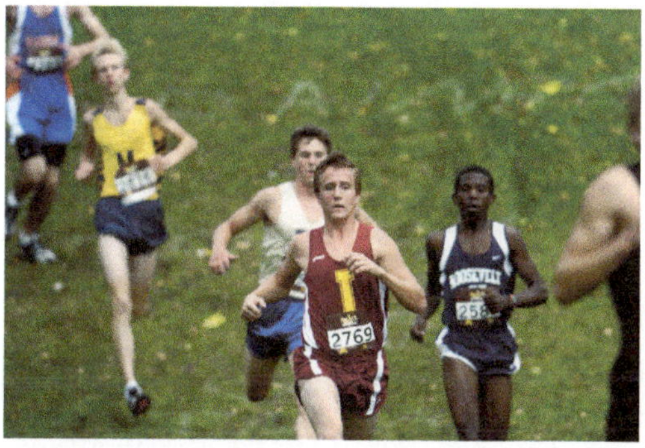

Competitors mid-race at a boys high school event in the United States

Cross country running is the most naturalistic of the sports in athletics as competitions take place on open-air courses over surfaces such as grass, woodland trails, and earth. It is both an individual and team sport, as runners are judged on an individual basis and a points scoring method is used for teams. Competitions are typically long distance races of 4 km (2.5 mi) or more which are usually held in autumn and winter. Cross country's most successful athletes often compete in long-distance track and road events as well.

The Crick Run in England in 1838 was the first recorded instance of an organised cross country competition. The sport gained popularity in British, then American schools in the 19th century and culminated in the creation of the first International Cross Country Championships in 1903. The annual IAAF World Cross Country Championships was inaugurated in 1973 and this remains the highest level of competition for the sport. A number of continental cross country competitions are held, with championships taking place in Asia, Europe, North America and South America. The sport has retained its status at the scholastic level, particularly in the United Kingdom and United States. At the professional level, the foremost competitions come under the banner of the IAAF Cross Country Permit Meetings.

While cross country competitions are no longer held at the Olympics, having featured in the athletics programme from 1912–1924, it has been present as one of the events within the modern pentathlon competition since the 1912 Summer Olympics. One variation on traditional cross country is mountain running, which incorporates significant uphill and/or downhill sections as an additional challenge to the course. Fell running and Orienteering are other competitive sports similar to cross country, although they feature an element of navigation which is absent from the set courses of cross country.

Racewalking

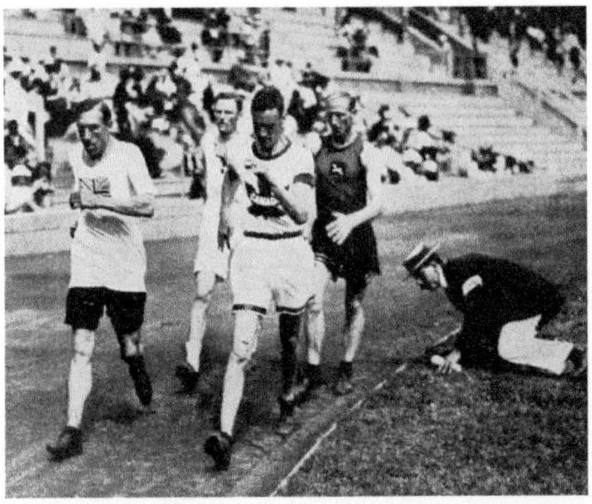

A track-side judge monitoring technique at the 1912 Summer Olympics in Stockholm, Sweden

Racewalking is a form of competitive walking that usually takes place on open-air roads, although running tracks are also occasionally used. Racewalking is the only sport in athletics in which judges monitor athletes on their technique. Racewalkers must always have a foot in contact with the ground and their advancing leg must be straightened, not bent at the knee – failure to follow these rules results in disqualification from the race.

Racewalking finds its roots in the sport of pedestrianism which emerged in the late 18th century in England. Spectators would gamble on the outcome of the walking competitions. The sport took on an endurance aspect and competitions were held over long distances or walkers would have to achieve a certain distance within a specified time frame, such as Centurion contests of walking 100 miles (160 km) within 24 hours. During this period, racewalking was frequently held on athletics tracks for ease of measurement, and the 1908 Summer Olympics in London saw the introduction of the 3500-metre and 10-mile walks. Racewalking was briefly dropped from the Olympic programme in 1928, but the men's 50 kilometres race walk has been held at every Olympic Games but one since 1932. The men's 20 kilometres race walk was added to the Olympic athletics schedule in 1956 and the women's event was first held in 1992. The most common events in modern competition are over 10 km, 20 km and 50 km on roads, although women's 3 km and men's 5 km are held on indoor tracks.

The highest level racewalking competitions occur at the IAAF World Championships in Athletics and at the Summer Olympics, although the sport also has its own separate major competition – the IAAF World Race Walking Cup – which has been held since 1961. The IAAF World Race Walking Challenge forms the primary seasonal competition – athletes earn points for their performances at ten selected racewalking competitions and the highest scoring walkers are entered into that year's IAAF Race Walking Challenge Final.

Categories

- Masters athletics, age groups spanning five years for athletes aged 35 and above
- Senior athletics, open class with no upper age limit but some limitations on younger people competing in endurance events
- Under 23, under the age of 23 years
- Junior, under the age of 20 years
- Youth, under the age of 18 years

Athletes with Disabilities

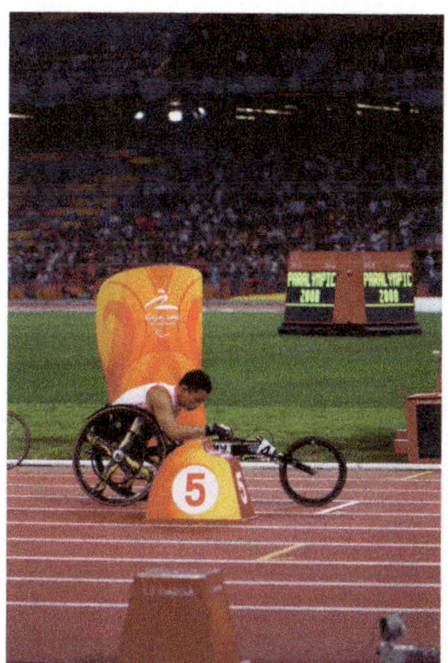

Competitor in a wheelchair race at the 2008 Summer Paralympics

Athletes with physical disabilities have competed at separate international events since 1952. The International Paralympic Committee governs the competitions in athletics, and hosts the Paralympic Games, which have continued since 1960.

Competitors at elite level competitions, are classified by disability, to arrange athletes with a similar disability in the same event. A classified T12 athlete for example, is a track athlete with a visual impairment.

- F – Field athletes
- T – Track athletes
- 11–13 – visual impairment. Compete with a sighted guide.
- 20 – Intellectual disability
- 31–38 – cerebral palsy
- 40–46 – amputation, and others (including athletes with dwarfism)
- 51–58 – Wheelchair

In wheelchair racing athletes compete in lightweight racing chairs. Most major marathons have wheelchair divisions and the elite racers consistently beat the runners on foot. The speed of wheel chair racers has caused difficulties for race organisers in properly staggering their start times compared to runners. A collision between Josh Cassidy (a wheelchair racer) and Tiki Gelana (a leading female marathoner) at the 2013 London Marathon brought the issue into the spotlight again.

Occasionally, athletes with a disability excel to compete with able bodied athletes. Legally blind Marla Runyan ran in the 2000 and 2004 Olympics and won a gold medal in the 1500 metres at the 1999 Pan American Games. Oscar Pistorius, a double amputee, has competed in the 2012 Olympics. At the 2011 World Championships Pistorius successfully made it to the 400 metres semi-final round and won a silver medal as part of South Africa's 4x400 metres relay team. In Masters athletics it is far more common to make an accommodation for athletes with a disability. Blind Ivy Granstrom set numerous Masters world records while being guided around the track.

Venues

Professional athletics almost exclusively takes place in one of three types of venue: stadiums, set courses on grass or woodland, and road-based courses. Such venues ensure that events take place in a relatively standardised manner, as well as improving the safety of athletes and enjoyment for spectators. At a more basic level, many forms of athletics demand very little in terms of venue requirements; almost any open space or area of field can provide a suitable venue for basic running, jumping and throwing competitions.

Track and Field Stadium

A standard outdoor track is in the shape of a stadium, 400 metres in length, and has at least eight lanes 1.22 m in width (small arenas might have six lanes). Older track facilities may have nonstandard track lengths, such as 440 yards (402.3 m; 1/4 mile) (common in the United States). Historically, tracks were covered by a dirt running surface. Modern All-weather running tracks are covered by a synthetic weather-resistant running surface, which typically consists of rubber (either black SBR or colored EPDM granules), bound by polyurethane or latex resins. Older tracks may be cinder-covered.

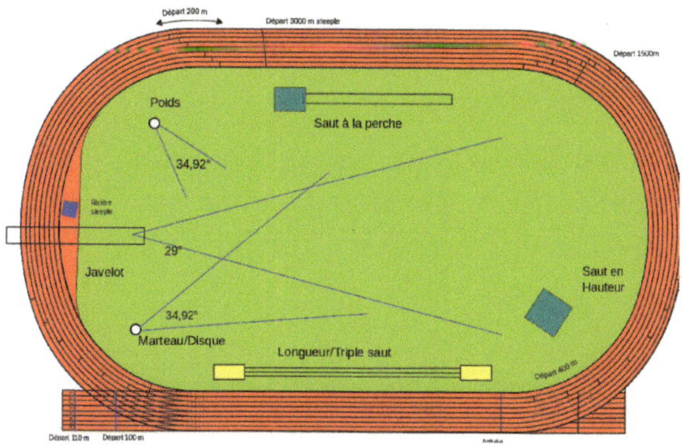

A typical layout of an outdoor track and field stadium

A standard indoor track is designed similarly to an outdoor track, but is only 200 metres in length and has between four and eight lanes, each with width between 0.90 m and 1.10 m. Often, the bends of an indoor track will be banked to compensate for the small turning radius. However, because of space limitations, indoor tracks may have other nonstandard lengths, such as 160-yard (146.3 m) indoor track at Madison Square Garden used for the Millrose Games. Because of space limitations, meetings held at indoor facilities do not hold many of athletics events typically contested outdoors.

Cross Country Courses

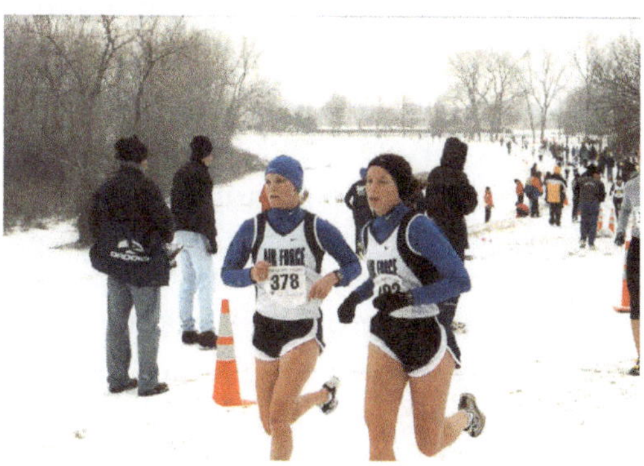

A cross country race taking place at a snowy park in the United States

There is no standardised form of cross country course and each venue is significantly defined by the environment it contains – some may be relatively flat and featureless, while others may be more challenging with natural obstacles, tight turns, and undulating ground. While a small number of purpose-built courses exist, the vast majority of cross country running courses are created by cordoning a specific area within any open natural land, typically a park, woodland or greenspace near a settlement.

At the elite and professional level, courses must be looped and each lap must be between 1750 m and 2000 m in length. Severe obstacles such as deep ditches, high barriers and thick undergrowth not normally present; the course should be able to be completed whilst remaining on foot throughout. In order to maintain the sport's distinction from road running, the usage of unnatural or macadamised surfaces is generally kept to a minimum or avoided entirely.

Because the majority of races take place on areas of grass, soil, mud or earth, weather conditions can significantly affect the difficulty of cross country courses, as snow and rain reduces traction and can create areas of standing water.

Road Courses

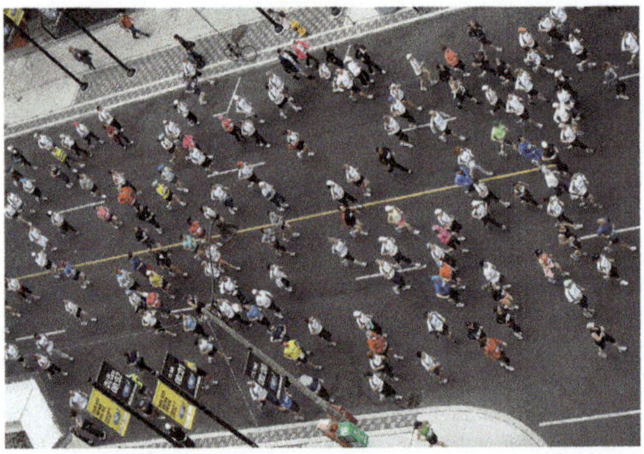

A typical road running course on the inner-city roads of Toronto

Thee surface of road races is highly important and the IAAF dictate that the courses must be along man-made roads, bicycle paths or footpaths. Courses set along major roads of cities are typical of road running events, and traffic is usually cordoned off from the area during the competition. While soft ground, such as grass, is generally avoided, races may start and finish on soft ground or within a track and field stadium. Road racing courses come in two primary types: looped and point-to-point. Courses may be measured and designed to cover a standardised distance, such as 10 km (6.2 mi), or they may simply follow a set route between two landmarks.

Road running courses over 5 km usually offer drinks or refreshment stations for runners at designated points alongside the course and medical professionals are present at the courses of major races due to the health risks involved with long-distance running.

Elite road walks are conducted on closed loop courses (usually loops of 2,000 or 2,500 meters). Refreshment stations are also present over long distance walking competitions, with drinks being available on every lap for races longer than 10 km.

Organizations

Since its foundation in 1912, the international governing body for athletics has been the International Association of Athletics Federations (IAAF). It was initially known as the

International Amateur Athletics Federation but changed later its name to reflect that the sport had moved away from amateurism towards professionalism in the late 1970s. The IAAF has 215 member nations and territories, which are divided into six continental areas (or area associations). The six association areas are for Asia, Africa, Europe, Oceania, North America and South America. The sports within athletics do not have their own independent governing bodies at either international or continental level, instead, all fall under the athletics authorities.

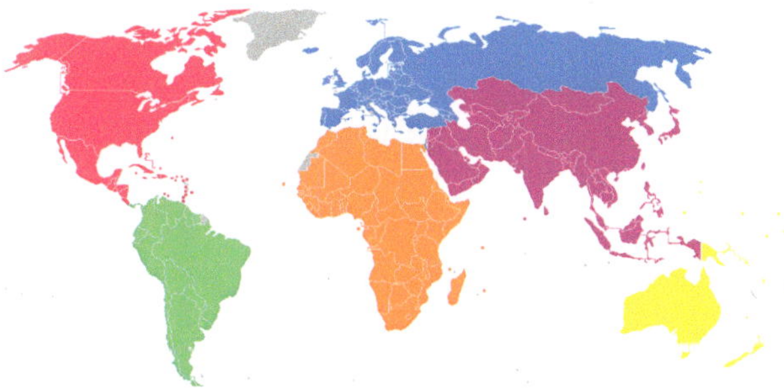

Map of the six continental federations of the IAAF

- AAA – Asian Athletics Association
- CAA – Confederation of African Athletics
- CONSUDATLE – South American Athletics Confederation
- NACACAA – North America, Central America and Caribbean Athletic Association
- EAA – European Athletics Association
- OAA – Oceania Athletics Association

National level athletics organisations are responsible for the regulation of the sport within their respective countries and most major competitions have some form of permit or approval from their national body.

Competitions

Athletics competitions can be broadly divided into three types: international championships, national championships, and annual meetings and races. Athletics at international championships, or Games, represent the pinnacle of competition within the sport, and they are contested between athletes representing their country or region. The organisation of these competitions is usually overseen by either a world, continental, or regional athletics governing body. Athletes gain entry into these competitions by earning selection from their national athletics governing body, which is generally done by assessing athletes via their past achievements or performances at a national selection event. National championships are annual competitions endorsed by a national governing body which serve the purpose of deciding the country's best athlete in each event. Annual one-day meetings and races form the most basic level of competition and are the most common format of athletics contests. These events are often invitational and are organised by sports organisations, sports promoters, or other institutions.

Competitions typically feature only one of the sports within athletics. However, major outdoor international athletics championships and athletics competitions held as part of multi-sport events usually feature a combination of track and field, road running and racewalking events.

International Championships

Olympic Games

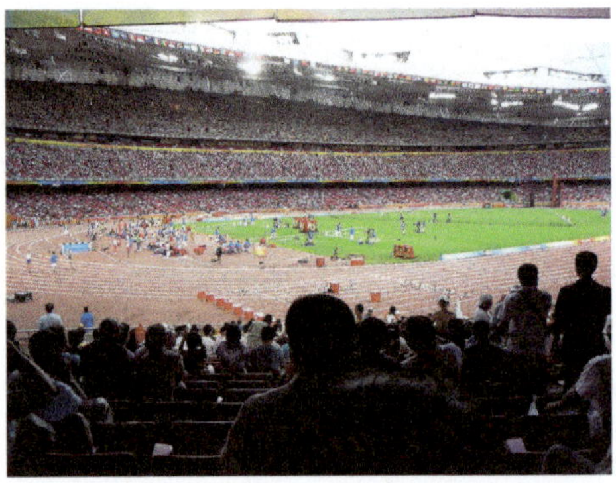

The athletics competition underway at the main stadium of the 2008 Summer Olympics

The modern Summer Olympics was the first event at which a global athletics competition took place. All the four major sports within athletics have featured in the Olympic athletics programme since its inception in 1896, although cross country has since been dropped. The Olympic competition is the most prestigious athletics contest, and many athletics events are among the most watched events at the Summer Olympics. A total of 47 athletics events are held at the Olympics, 24 for men and 23 for women (as of London 2012). The events within the men's and women's programmes are either identical or have a similar equivalent, with the sole exception being that men contest the 50 km race walk.

Paralympic Games

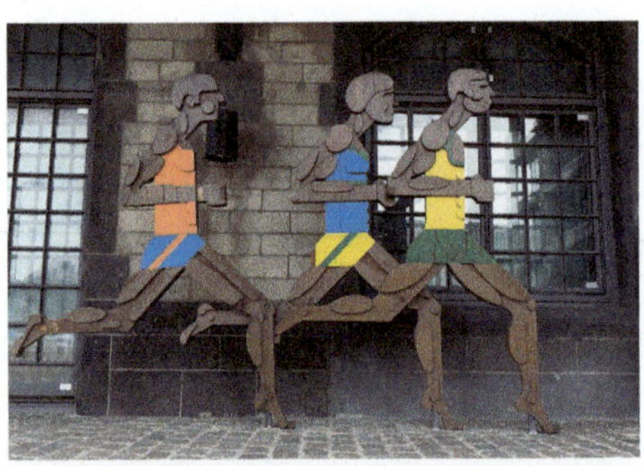

Athletics Figure before Olympic Museum Cologne

The Summer Paralympics include athletes with a physical disability. Track and field, and road events have featured in the Paralympic athletics programme since its inception in 1960. The Paralympic competition is the most prestigious athletics contest where athletes with a physical disability compete.

Athletics at the Paralympic Games also include wheelchair racing where athletes compete in lightweight racing chairs. Athletes with a visual impairment compete with a sighted guide. At the 2012 Summer Paralympics in London, for the first time at an international athletics event, the guides received medals, such as the pilots in cycling, and the guides at the Paralympic Winter Games have done for a while.

World Championships

The IAAF World Championships in Athletics is the primary global athletics championships held by IAAF. The biennial competition was first held in 1983 and now features an event programme which is identical to the Olympics. Thus, road running, racewalking and track and field are the sports which feature at the competition. Cross country running has its own discrete global championships – the IAAF World Cross Country Championships – which has been held annually since 1973. The IAAF World Indoor Championships in Athletics is a biennial athletics championships which features solely indoor track and field events. The foremost separate road running event is the annual IAAF World Half Marathon Championships (formerly World Road Running Championships). While not having official world championship status, the biennial IAAF World Race Walking Cup fulfils a similar role for the sport of racewalking. Outdoor track and field is the only sport in athletics that does not have a its own distinct global championship which is separate from other types of athletics, although the IAAF Continental Cup (a quadrennial competition between continental teams) is composed entirely of outdoor track and field events.

Other world championships include the IAAF World Junior and World Youth Championships in Athletics, which are for athletes under-19 and under-17, respectively. World Masters Athletics conducts the World Masters Athletics Championships for athletes in 5-year age divisions over the age of 35. The now defunct IAAF World Road Relay Championships served as the global event for Ekiden marathon relay races.

Elite athletes with a physical disability compete at the IPC Athletics World Championships (to be renamed the World Para Athletics Championships as of the next edition in 2017) and at the Commonwealth Games.

Commonwealth Games

Athletics is one of the sports at the quadrennial Commonwealth Games competition. It has been a Commonwealth Games sport since the inaugural edition of the event's precursor, the 1930 British Empire Games. It is a core sport and must be included in the sporting programme of each edition of the Games.

Universiade

Athletics is one of the sports at the biennial summer Universiade competition. It has been one of the event's competed sports since the inaugural edition.

Culture and Media

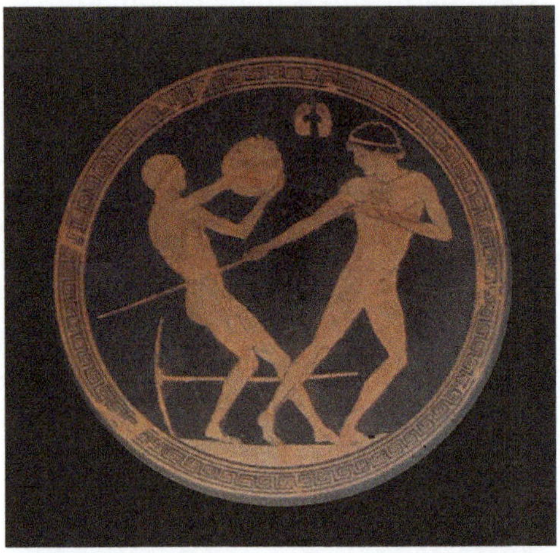

Ancient Greek pottery showing the javelin and the discus throw

Athletics, and its athletes in particular, has been artistically depicted since ancient times – one of the surviving instances include runners and high jumpers in the motifs of Ancient Egyptian tombs dating from 2250 BCE. Athletics was much respected in Ancient Greece and the events within the ancient pentathlon provided inspiration for large statues such as the Discobolus and Discophoros, and for motifs on countless vase and pottery works. Aristotle discussed the significance of the pentathlon in his treatise *Rhetoric* and reflected on the athlete aesthetic of the period: "a body capable of enduring all efforts, either of the racecourse or of bodily strength...This is why the athletes in the pentathlon are most beautiful".

Films about athletics are overwhelmingly focused on running events: the 1962 film *The Loneliness of the Long Distance Runner* (based on the book of the same name) explores cross country running as a means of escape. *Chariots of Fire*, perhaps one of the most well-known athletics films, is a fictionalised account of Eric Liddell and Harold Abrahams's chase for sprint gold medals at the 1924 Olympics. Track and field has been the subject of American films such as *Personal Best* (1981) and *Across the Tracks* (1991). Biopics are found within the genre, including *Prefontaine* (regarding Steve Prefontaine) and *Jim Thorpe – All-American* (1951) featuring Burt Lancaster as Thorpe. Documentaries are also common with examples such as 2007 film *Spirit of the Marathon*, which follows runners' preparations for the 2005 Chicago Marathon.

Books on the subject are predominantly non-fiction, and tend towards the forms of training manuals and historical accounts of athletics. The story of the four-minute mile has been a particularly popular subject, spawning books such as *The Perfect Mile* and *3:59.4: The Quest to Break the Four Minute Mile*.

Athletics journalism has spawned a number of dedicated periodicals including *Athletics Weekly* and *Race Walking Record*, both of which were first published in England in the early 1940s, and *Track & Field News* which was first published in the United States in 1948. *Runner's World* has been in print since 1966 and the *Track & Field Magazine of Japan* (*Rikujyo Kyogi Magazine*) is another long-running publication.

Athletics events have been selected as a main motif in numerous collectors' coins. One of the recent samples is the €10 Greek Running commemorative coin, minted in 2003 to commemorate the 2004 Summer Olympics. In the obverse of the coin, a modern athlete figure appears in the foreground, shown in the starting position, while in the background two ancient runners are carved in a manner that gives the appearance of a coin that is "worn" by time. This scene originally appeared on a black-figure vase of the 6th century BCE.

References

- Sansone, David (1992). Greek athletics and the genesis of sport, p.72. University of California Press. ISBN 0-520-08095-5
- "Archived copy: The Effects of Mental Imagery on Athletic Performance". Archived from the original on 2011-06-07. Retrieved 2011-06-26
- Delforge, G.D.; Behnke, R.S. (1999). "The History and Evolution of Athletic Training Education in the United States". Journal of Athletic Training. 34 (1): 53–61
- "Archived copy:Basic Concepts in Sports Biomechanics". Archived from the original on 2011-10-28. Retrieved 2011-10-27
- "Commission on Accreditation of Athletic Training Education: Overview of the Commission". Retrieved 11 May 2012

2

Athletic Training and Exercises

Endurance training is the training undergone by athletes to increase their strength. Endurance training can be divided into two categories, general and specific. Strength training, cross-training and physical exercise are some of the exercises discussed in the following section. The major components of athletic training and performance are discussed in this chapter.

Endurance Training

Endurance training is the act of exercising to increase endurance. The term endurance training generally refers to training the aerobic system as opposed to anaerobic. The need for endurance in sports is often predicated as the need of cardiovascular and simple muscular endurance, but the issue of endurance is far more complex. Endurance can be divided into two categories including: general endurance and specific endurance. It can be shown that endurance in sport is closely tied to the execution of skill and technique. A well conditioned athlete can be defined as, the athlete who executes his or her technique consistently and effectively with the least effort.

Endurance in Sports

Endurance training is essential for a variety of endurance sports. A notable example is distance running events (800 meters upwards to marathon and ultra-marathon) with the required degree of endurance training increasing with race distance. Two other popular examples are cycling (particularly road cycling) and competitive swimming. These three endurance sports are combined in triathlon. Other endurance sports for which extensive amounts of endurance trained include rowing and cross country skiing. Athletes can also undergo endurance training when their sport may not necessarily be an endurance sport in the whole sense but may still demand some endurance. For instance aerobic endurance is necessary (to varying extents) in racket sports, football, rugby, martial arts, basketball and cricket. Endurance exercise tends to be popular with non-athletes for the purpose of increasing general fitness or burning more calories to increase weight loss potential.

Physiological Effects

Long-term endurance training induces many physiological adaptations both centrally and peripherally mediated. Central cardiovascular adaptations include decreased heart rate, increased stroke volume of the heart, increased blood plasma, without any major changes in red blood cell count, which reduces blood viscosity and increased cardiac output as well as total mitochondrial volume in the muscle fibers used in the training (i.e. the thigh muscles in runners will have more mitochondria than the thigh muscles of swimmers). Mitochondria increase in both number and size and there are similar increases in myoglobin and oxidative enzymes. Adaptations of the peripheral include capillarization, that is an increase in the surface area that both the venous and arterial capillaries supply. This also allows for increased heat dissipation during strenuous exercise. The muscles heighten their glycogen and fat storing capabilities in endurance athletes in order to increase the length in time in which they can perform work. Endurance training primarily work the slow twitch (type 1) fibers and develop such fibers in their efficiency and resistance to fatigue. Catabolism also improves increasing the athletes capacity to use fat and glycogen stores as an energy source. These metabolic processes are known as glycogenolysis, glycolysis and lipolysis. There is higher efficiency in oxygen transport and distribution. In recent years it has been recognized that oxidative enzymes such as succinate dehydrogenase (SDH) that enable mitochondria to break down nutrients to form ATP increase by 2.5 times in well trained endurance athletes In addition to SDH, myoglobin increases by 75-80% in well trained endurance athletes.

Risks of Excessive Endurance Training

The potential for negative health effects from long-term, high-volume endurance training have begun to emerge in the scientific literature in recent years. The known risks are primarily associated with training for and participation in extreme endurance events, and affect the cardiovascular system through adverse structural remodeling of the heart and the associated arteries, with heart-rhythm abnormalities perhaps being the most common resulting symptom.

Endurance Exercise can also reduce testosterone levels.

Methods and Training Plans

Common methods for training include periodization, intervals, hard easy, long slow distance, and in recent years high-intensity interval training. The periodization method is very common and was accredited to Tudor Bompa and consists of blocks of time, generally 4–12 weeks each. The blocks are called preparation, base, build and race. The goal of a structured training program with periodization is to bring the athlete into peak fitness at the time of a big race or event. Preparation as the name suggests lays the groundwork for heavier work to follow. For a runner contemplating a competitive marathon the preparation phase might consist of easier runs of 1–4 miles 3-4 times per week and including 2–3 days of core strengthening. In the base phase the athlete now works on building cardiovascular endurance by having several long runs staying in heart rate zone 1-2 every week and each week adding slightly more mileage (using 10% rule for safely increasing the mileage). Core strengthening is continued in the base period. Once the base phase is complete and the athlete has sufficient endurance, the build period is needed to give the athlete the ability to hold a faster pace for the race duration. The build phase is where duration of runs is traded for intensity or heart rate zones 3-5. An easy method to obtain intensity is interval training and interval training starts to happen in the build phase. Through interval training during the build phase the athlete can achieve higher lactate threshold and in some athletes VO2 max is increased. Because interval training is demanding on the body, a professional coach should be consulted. In the very least the athlete should do a warm up and active stretching before the interval session and static stretch or yoga after hard interval sessions. It is also advisable to have days of rest or easy workouts the day after interval sessions. Finally the race phase of the periodization approach is where the duration of the workouts decreases but intense workouts remain so as to keep the high lactate threshold that was gained in the build phase. In Ironman training, the race phase is where a long "taper" occurs of up to 4 weeks for highly trained Ironman racers. A final phase is designated transition and is a period of time, where the body is allowed to recover from the hard race effort and some maintenance endurance training is performed so the high fitness level attained in the previous periods will not be lost.

Traditionally, strength training (the performance of exercises with resistance or added weight) was not deemed appropriate for endurance athletes due to potential interference in the adaptive response to the endurance elements of an athlete's training plan. There were also misconceptions regarding the addition of excess body mass through muscle hypertrophy (growth) associated with strength training, which could negatively effect endurance performance by increasing the amount of work required to be completed by the athlete. However, more recent and comprehensive research has proved that short-term (8 weeks) strength training in addition to endurance training is beneficial for endurance performance, particularly long-distance running.

Devices to Assess Endurance Fitness

The heart rate monitor is one of the relatively easy methods to assess fitness in endurance athletes. By comparing heart rate over time fitness gains can be observed when the heart rate decreases for running or cycling at a given speed. In cycling the effect of wind on the cyclists speed is difficult to subtract out and so many cyclists now use power meters built into their bicycles. The power meter allows the athlete to actually measure power output over a set duration or course and allows direct comparison of fitness progression. In the 2008 Olympics Michael Phelps was aided by repeated lactate threshold measurement. This allowed his coaches to fine tune his training program so that he could recover between swim events that were sometimes several minutes apart. Much similar to blood glucose for diabetes, lower priced lactate measurement devices are now available but in general the lactate measurement approach is still the domain of the professional coach and elite athlete.

Strength Training

Strength training is a type of physical exercise specializing in the use of resistance to induce muscular contraction which builds the strength, anaerobic endurancc, and size of skeletal muscles.

When properly performed, strength training can provide significant functional benefits and improvement in overall health and well-being, including increased bone, muscle, tendon and ligament strength and toughness, improved joint function, reduced potential for injury, increased bone density, increased metabolism, increased fitness, improved cardiac function, and improved lipoprotein lipid profiles, including elevated HDL ("good") cholesterol. Training commonly uses the technique of progressively increasing the force output of the muscle through incremental weight increases and uses a variety of exercises and types of equipment to target specific muscle groups. Strength training is primarily an anaerobic activity, although some proponents have adapted it to provide the benefits of aerobic exercise through circuit training.

Strength training is typically associated with the production of lactate, which is a limiting factor of exercise performance. Regular endurance exercise leads to adaptations in skeletal muscle which can prevent lactate levels from rising during strength training. This is mediated via activation of PGC-1alpha which alter the LDH (lactate dehydrogenase) isoenzyme complex composition and decreases the activity of the lactate generating enzyme LDHA, while increasing the activity of the lactate metabolizing enzyme LDHB.

Sports where strength training is central are bodybuilding, weightlifting, powerlifting, strongman, Highland games, shotput, discus throw, and javelin throw. Many other sports use strength training as part of their training regimen, notably tennis, American football, wrestling, track and field, rowing, lacrosse, basketball, pole dancing, hockey, professional wrestling, rugby union, rugby league and soccer. Strength training for other sports and physical activities is becoming increasingly popular.

Uses

The benefits of weight training include greater muscular strength, improved muscle tone and appearance, increased endurance and enhanced bone density.

Increased Physical Attractiveness

Many people take up weight training to improve their physical attractiveness. There is evidence that a body type consisting of broad shoulders and a narrow waist, attainable through strength training, is the most physically attractive male attribute according to women participating in the research. Most men can develop substantial muscles; most women lack the testosterone to do it, but they can develop a firm, "toned" physique, and they can increase their strength by the same proportion as that achieved by men (but usually from a significantly lower starting point). An individual's genetic make-up dictates the response to weight training stimuli to a significant extent, training can not exceed a muscle's intrinsic genetically determined qualities, but clearly polymorphic expression of Myosin heavy chains is possible.

Workouts elevate metabolism for up to 14 hours following 45-minutes of vigorous exercise.

Increased General Physical Health

Strength training also provides functional benefits. Stronger muscles improve posture, provide better support for joints, and reduce the risk of injury from everyday activities. Older people who take up weight training can prevent some of the loss of muscle tissue that normally accompanies aging—and even regain some functional strength—and by doing so become less frail. They may be able to avoid some types of physical disability. Weight-bearing exercise also helps to prevent osteoporosis and to improve bone strength in those with osteoporosis. The benefits of weight training for older people have been confirmed by studies of people who began engaging in it even in their 80s and 90s.

Though strength training can stimulate the cardiovascular system, many exercise physiologists, based on their observation of maximal oxygen uptake, argue that aerobics training is a better cardiovascular stimulus. Central catheter monitoring during resistance training reveals increased cardiac output, suggesting that strength training shows potential for cardiovascular exercise. However, a 2007 meta-analysis found that, though aerobic training is an effective therapy for heart failure patients, combined aerobic and strength training is ineffective.

Strength training may be important to metabolic and cardiovascular health. Recent evidence suggests that resistance training may reduce metabolic and cardiovascular disease risk. Overweight individuals with high strength fitness exhibit metabolic/cardiovascular risk profiles similar to normal-weight, fit individuals rather than overweight unfit individuals.

For Rehabilitation or to Address an Impairment

For many people in rehabilitation or with an acquired disability, such as following stroke or orthopaedic surgery, strength training for weak muscles is a key factor to optimise recovery. For people with such a health condition, their strength training is likely to need to be designed by an appropriate health professional, such as a physiotherapist or an occupational therapist.

Increased Sports Performance

Stronger muscles improve performance in a variety of sports. Sport-specific training routines are used by many competitors. These often specify that the speed of muscle contraction during weight training should be the same as that of the particular sport.

For the Pleasure of the Activity

One side effect of any intense exercise is increased levels of dopamine, serotonin, and norepinephrine, which can help to improve mood and counter feelings of depression.

Developing research has demonstrated that many of the benefits of exercise are mediated through the role of skeletal muscle as an endocrine organ. That is, contracting muscles release multiple substances known as myokines which promote the growth of new tissue, tissue repair, and various anti-inflammatory functions, which in turn reduce the risk of developing various inflammatory diseases.

Technique

The basic principles of strength training involve a manipulation of the number of repetitions (reps), sets, tempo, exercises and force to cause desired changes in strength, endurance or size by overloading of a group of muscles. The specific combinations of reps, sets, exercises, resistance and force depend on the purpose of the individual performing the exercise: to gain size and strength multiple (4+) sets with fewer reps must be performed using more force. A wide spectrum of regimens can be adopted to achieve different results, but the classic formula recommended by the American College of Sports Medicine reads as follows:

- 8 to 12 repetitions of a resistance training exercise for each major muscle group at an intensity of 40% to 80% of a one-repetition max (RM) depending on the training level of the participant.
- Two to three minutes of rest is recommended between exercise sets to allow for proper recovery.
- Two to four sets are recommended for each muscle group.

Typically failure to use good form during a training set can result in injury or an inability to meet training goals – since the desired muscle group is not challenged sufficiently, the threshold of overload is never reached and the muscle does not gain in strength. There are cases when cheating is beneficial, as is the case where weaker groups become the weak link in the chain and the target muscles are never fully exercised as a result.

The benefits of strength training include increased muscle, tendon and ligament strength, bone density, flexibility, tone, metabolic rate and postural support.

Terminology

Strength training has a variety of specialized terms used to describe parameters of strength training:

- Exercise – different movements which involve rotating joints in specific patterns to challenge muscles in different ways.
- Form – each exercise has a specific form, a topography of movement designed to maximize safety and muscle strength gains.
- Rep – short for repetition, a rep is a single cycle of lifting and lowering a weight in a controlled manner, moving through the form of the exercise.
- Set – a set consists of several repetitions performed one after another with no break between them with the number of reps per set and sets per exercise depending on the goal of the individual. The number of repetitions one can perform at a certain weight is called the Rep Maximum (RM). For example, if one could perform ten reps at 75 lbs, then their RM for that weight would be 10RM. 1RM is therefore the maximum weight that someone can lift in a given exercise – i.e. a weight that they can only lift once without a break.
- Tempo – the speed with which an exercise is performed; the tempo of a movement has implications for the weight that can be moved and the effects on the muscle.

Realization of Training Goals

For developing endurance, gradual increases in volume and gradual decreases in intensity is the most effective program. Sets of thirteen to twenty repetitions develop anaerobic endurance, with some increases to muscle size and limited impact on strength.

It has been shown that for beginners, multiple-set training offers minimal benefits over single-set training with respect to either strength gain or muscle mass increase, but for the experienced athlete multiple-set systems are required for optimal progress. However, one study shows that for leg muscles, three sets are more effective than one set.

Beginning weight-trainers are in the process of training the neurological aspects of strength, the ability of the brain to generate a rate of neuronal action potentials that will produce a muscular contraction that is close to the maximum of the muscle's potential.

Variable	Training goal				
	Strength	Power	Hypertrophy	Endurance	Speed
Load (% of 1RM)	90–80	60–45	80–60	60–40	30
Reps per set	1–5	1–5	6–12	13–60	1–5
Sets per exercise	4–7	3–5	4–8	2–4	3–5
Rest between sets (mins)	2–6	2–6	2–3	1–2	2–5
Duration (seconds per set)	5–10	4–8	20–60	80–150	20–40

Speed per rep (% of max)	60–100	90–100	60–90	60–80	100
Training sessions per week	3–6	3–6	5–7	8–14	3–6

Weights for each exercise should be chosen so that the desired number of repetitions can just be achieved.

Progressive Overload

In one common method, weight training uses the principle of progressive overload, in which the muscles are overloaded by attempting to lift at least as much weight as they are capable. They respond by growing larger and stronger. This procedure is repeated with progressively heavier weights as the practitioner gains strength and endurance.

However, performing exercises at the absolute limit of one's strength (known as one rep max lifts) is considered too risky for all but the most experienced practitioners. Moreover, most individuals wish to develop a combination of strength, endurance and muscle size. One repetition sets are not well suited to these aims. Practitioners therefore lift lighter (sub-maximal) weights, with more repetitions, to fatigue the muscle and all fibres within that muscle as required by the progressive overload principle.

Commonly, each exercise is continued to the point of momentary muscular failure. Contrary to widespread belief, this is not the point at which the individual thinks they cannot complete any more repetitions, but rather the first repetition that fails due to inadequate muscular strength. Training to failure is a controversial topic with some advocating training to failure on all sets while others believe that this will lead to overtraining, and suggest training to failure only on the last set of an exercise. Some practitioners recommend finishing a set of repetitions just before reaching a personal maximum at a given time. Adrenaline and other hormones may promote additional intensity by stimulating the body to lift additional weight (as well as the neuro-muscular stimulations that happen when in "fight-or-flight" mode, as the body activates more muscle fibres), so getting "psyched up" before a workout can increase the maximum weight lifted.

Weight training can be a very effective form of strength training because exercises can be chosen, and weights precisely adjusted, to safely exhaust each individual muscle group after the specific numbers of sets and repetitions that have been found to be the most effective for the individual. Other strength training exercises lack the flexibility and precision that weights offer.

Split Training

Split training involves working no more than three muscle groups or body parts per day, instead spreading the training of specific body parts throughout a training cycle of several days. It is commonly used by more advanced practitioners due to the logistics involved in training all muscle groups maximally. Training all the muscles in the body individually through their full range of motion in a single day is generally not considered possible due to caloric and time constraints. Split training involves fully exhausting individual muscle groups during a workout, then allowing several days for the muscle to fully recover. Muscles are worked roughly twice per week and allowed roughly 72 hours to recover. Recovery of certain muscle groups is usually achieved on days while training other groups, i.e. a 7-day week can consist of a practitioner training trapezius, side shoulders and upper shoulders to exhaustion on one day, the following day the arms to exhaustion, the day after that the rear, front shoulders and back, the day after that the chest. In this way all mentioned muscle groups are allowed the necessary recovery.

Intensity, Volume and Frequency

Three important variables of strength training are intensity, volume, and frequency. Intensity refers to the amount of work required to achieve the activity, and is proportional to the mass of the weights being lifted. Volume refers to the number of muscles worked, exercises, sets and reps during a single session. Frequency refers to how many training sessions are performed per week.

These variables are important because they are all mutually conflicting, as the muscle only has so much strength and endurance, and takes time to recover due to microtrauma. Increasing one by any significant amount necessitates the decrease of the other two, e.g. increasing weight means a reduction of reps, and will require more recovery time and therefore fewer workouts per week. Trying to push too much intensity, volume and frequency will result in overtraining, and eventually lead to injury and other health issues such as chronic soreness and general lethargy, illness or even acute trauma such as avulsion fractures. A high-medium-low formula can be used to avoid overtraining, with either intensity, volume, or frequency being high, one of the others being medium, and the other being low. One example of this training strategy can be found in the following chart:

Type	High	Med	Low
Intensity (% of 1RM)	80–100%	50–70%	10–40%
Volume (per muscle)	1 exercise	2 exercises	3+ exercises
Sets	1 set	2–3 sets	4+ sets
Reps	1–6 reps	8–15 reps	20+ reps
Session frequency	1 p/w	2–3 p/w	4+ p/w

A common training strategy is to set the volume and frequency the same each week (e.g. training 3 times per week, with 2 sets of 12 reps each workout), and steadily increase the intensity (weight) on a weekly basis. However, to maximize progress to specific goals, individual programs may require different manipulations, such as decreasing the weight, and increase volume or frequency.

Making program alterations on a daily basis (daily undulating periodization) seems to be more efficient in eliciting strength gains than doing so every 4 weeks (linear periodization), but for beginners there are no differences between different periodization models.

Periodization

There are many complicated definitions for periodization, but the term simply means the division of the overall training program into periods which accomplish different goals.

Periodization is the modulating of volume, intensity, and frequency over time, to both stimulate gains and allow recovery.

In some programs for example; volume is decreased during a training cycle while intensity is increased. In this template, a lifter would begin a training cycle with a higher rep range than he will finish with.

For this example, the lifter has a 1 rep max of 225 lb:

Week	Set 1	Set 2	Set 3	Set 4	Set 5	Volume Lbs.	% Exertion(Last Set)	% of 1 Rep Max(Last Set)
1	125 lb x 8reps	130 lb x 8reps	135 lb x 8reps	140 lb x 8reps	145 lb x 8reps	5,400	78%	64%
2	135 lb x 7reps	140 lb x 7reps	145 lb x 7reps	150 lb x 7reps	155 lb x 7reps	5,075	81%	69%
3	145 lb x 6reps	150 lb x 6reps	155 lb x 6reps	160 lb x 6reps	165 lb x 6reps	4,650	84%	73%
4	155 lb x 5reps	160 lb x 5reps	165 lb x 5reps	170 lb x 5reps	175 lb x 5reps	4,125	87%	78%
5	165 lb x 4reps	170 lb x 4reps	175 lb x 4reps	180 lb x 4reps	185 lb x 4reps	3,500	90%	82%
6	175 lb x 3reps	180 lb x 3reps	185 lb x 3reps	190 lb x 3reps	195 lb x 3reps	2,775	92%	87%

This is an example of periodization where the number of repetitions decreases while the weight increases.

Practice of Weight Training

Methods and Equipment

There are many methods of strength training. Examples include weight training, circuit training, isometric exercise, gymnastics, plyometrics, Parkour, yoga, Pilates, Super Slow.

Strength training may be done with minimal or no equipment, for instance bodyweight exercises. Equipment used for strength training includes barbells and dumbbells, weight machines and other exercise machines, weighted clothing, resistance bands, gymnastics apparatus, Swiss balls, wobble boards, indian clubs, pneumatic exercise equipment, hydraulic exercise equipment.

Aerobic Exercise Versus Anaerobic Exercise

Strength training exercise is primarily anaerobic. Even while training at a lower intensity (training loads of ~20-RM), anaerobic glycolysis is still the major source of power, although aerobic metabolism makes a small contribution. Weight training is commonly perceived as anaerobic exercise, because one of the more common goals is to increase strength by lifting heavy weights. Other goals such as rehabilitation, weight loss, body shaping, and bodybuilding often use lower weights, adding aerobic character to the exercise.

Except in the extremes, a muscle will fire fibres of both the aerobic or anaerobic types on any given exercise, in varying ratio depending on the load on the intensity of the contraction. This is known as the energy system continuum. At higher loads, the muscle will recruit all muscle fibres possible, both anaerobic ("fast-twitch") and aerobic ("slow-twitch"), in order to generate the most force. However, at maximum load, the anaerobic processes contract so forcefully that the aerobic fibers are completely shut out, and all work is done by the anaerobic processes. Because the anaerobic muscle fibre uses its fuel faster than the blood and intracellular restorative cycles can resupply it, the maximum number of repetitions is limited. In the aerobic regime, the blood and intracellular processes can maintain a supply of fuel and oxygen, and continual repetition of the motion will not cause the muscle to fail.

Circuit weight training is a form of exercise that uses a number of weight training exercise sets separated by short intervals. The cardiovascular effort to recover from each set serves a function similar to an aerobic exercise, but this is not the same as saying that a weight training set is itself an aerobic process.

Exercises for Specific Muscle Groups

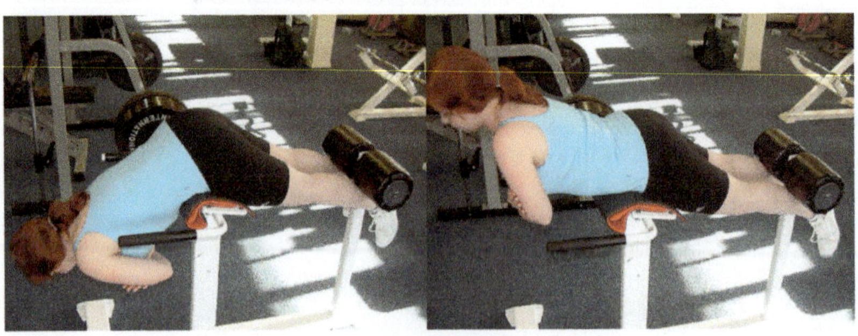

A *back extension*

Weight trainers commonly divide the body's individual muscles into ten major muscle groups. These do not include the hip, neck and forearm muscles, which are rarely trained in isolation. The most common exercises for these muscle groups are listed below.

The sequence shown below is one possible way to order the exercises. The large muscles of the lower body are normally trained before the smaller muscles of the upper body, because these first exercises require more mental and physical energy. The core muscles of the torso are trained before the shoulder and arm muscles that assist them. Exercises often alternate between "pushing" and "pulling" movements to allow their specific supporting muscles time to recover. The stabilizing muscles in the waist should be trained last.

Advanced Techniques

A number of techniques have been developed to make weight training exercises more intense, and thereby potentially increase the rate of progress. Many weight lifters use these techniques to bring themselves past a plateau, a duration where a weightlifter may be unable to do more lifting repetitions, sets, or use higher weight resistance.

Sct Structure

Drop sets

> Drop sets do not end at the point of momentary muscular failure, but continue with progressively lighter weights.

Pyramid sets

> Pyramid sets are weight training sets in which the progression is from lighter weights with a greater number of repetitions in the first set, to heavier weights with fewer repetitions in subsequent sets.

A reverse pyramid is the opposite in which the heavier weights are used at the beginning and progressively lightened.

Burnouts

> Burnouts combine pyramids and drop sets, working up to higher weights with low reps and then back down to lower weights and high reps.

Diminishing set

> The diminishing set method is where a weight is chosen that can be lifted for 20 reps in one set, and then 70 repetitions are performed in as few sets as possible.

Rest-pause (heavy singles)

> Rest-pause heavy singles are performed at or near 1RM, with ten to twenty seconds of rest between each lift. The lift is repeated six to eight times. It is generally recommended to use this method infrequently.

Giant set

The Giant set, is a form of training that targets one muscle group (e.g. the triceps) with four separate exercises performed in quick succession, often to failure and sometimes with the reduction of weight halfway through a set once muscle fatigue sets in. This form of intense training 'shocks' the muscles and as such, is usually performed by experienced trainers and should be used infrequently.

Combined Sets

Supersets

Supersets combine two or more exercises with similar motions to maximize the amount of work of an individual muscle or group of muscles. The exercises are performed with no rest period between the exercises. An example would be doing bench press, which predominantly works the pectoralis and triceps muscles, and then moving to an exercise that works just the triceps such as the triceps extension or the pushdown.

Push-pull supersets

Push-pull supersets are similar to regular supersets, but exercises are chosen which work opposing muscle groups. This is especially popular when applied to arm exercises, for example by combining biceps curls with the triceps pushdown. Other examples include the shoulder press and lat pulldown combination, and the bench press and wide grip row combination.

Pre-exhaustion

Pre-exhaustion combines an isolation exercise with a compound exercise for the same muscle group. The isolation exercise first exhausts the muscle group, and then the compound exercise uses the muscle group's supporting muscles to push it further than would otherwise be possible. For example, the triceps muscles normally help the pectorals perform their function. But in the "bench press" the weaker triceps often fails first, which limits the impact on the pectorals. By preceding the bench press with the pec fly, the pectorals can be pre-exhausted so that both muscles fail at the same time, and both benefit equally from the exercise.

Breakdowns

Breakdowns were developed by Fredrick Hatfield and Mike Quinn to work the different types of muscle fibers for maximum stimulation. Three different exercises that work the same muscle group are selected, and used for a superset. The first exercise uses a heavy weight (~85% of 1 rep max) for around five reps, the second a medium weight (~70% of 1 rep max) for around twelve reps, and finally the third exercise is performed with a light weight (~50% of 1 rep max) for twenty to thirty reps, or even lighter (~40% of 1 rep max) for forty or more reps. (Going to failure is discouraged.) The entire superset is performed three times.

Beyond Failure

Forced reps

Forced reps occur after momentary muscular failure. An assistant provides just enough help to get the weight trainer past the sticking point of the exercise, and allow further repetitions to be completed. Weight trainers often do this when they are spotting their exercise partner. With some exercises forced reps can be done without a training partner. For example, with one-arm *biceps curls* the other arm can be used to assist the arm that is being trained.

Cheat reps

Cheating is a deliberate compromise of form to maximize reps. Cheating has the advantage that it can be done without a training partner, but compromises safety. A typical example of cheat reps occurs during biceps curls when, beginning with the load at the waist, the exerciser swings the barbell or dumbbell forward and up during the concentric phase utilizing momentum to assist their bicep muscles in moving the load to a shortened muscle position. Momentum assistance during the concentric phase allows them to move greater loads during the more difficult concentric phase. The objective can be to position greater loads of resistance to the biceps in preparation of performing the eccentric phase than the more difficult concentric phase would otherwise allow. Replacing a typical function of a training partner with a solo exerciser performing cheat reps facilitates forced reps or negative reps when training alone.

Rest-pause (post-failure)

After a normal set of 6–8 reps (to failure), the weight is re-racked and the trainer takes 10–15 deep breaths, and then performs one more repetition. This process can be repeated for two further repetitions. The twenty-rep squat is another, similar approach, in that it follows a 12–15 rep set of squats with individual rest-pause reps, up to a total of 20 reps.

Weight stripping a.k.a. Number Setting

Weight stripping is a technique used after failure with a normal resistance in certain exercises, particularly with easily adjustable machines, whereby the weight trainer or a partner gradually reduces the resistance after a full set is taken to failure. With each reduction in resistance, as many possible reps are completed and the resistance is then reduced again. This is continued until the resistance is approximately half the original resistance.

Negative reps

Negative reps are performed with much heavier weights. Assistants lift the weight, and then the weight trainer attempts to resist its downward progress through an eccentric contraction. Alternatively, an individual can use an exercise machine for negatives by lifting the weight with both arms or legs, and then lowering it with only one. Or they can simply lower weights more slowly than they lift them: for example, by taking two seconds to lift each weight and four seconds to lower it.

Partial reps

Partial reps, as the name implies, involves movement through only part of the normal path of an exercise. Partial reps can be performed with heavier weights. Usually, only the easiest part of the repetition is attempted.

Burns

Burns involve mixing partial reps into a set of full range reps in order to increase intensity. The partials can be performed at any part of the exercise movement, depending on what works best for the particular exercise. Also, the partials can either be added after the end of a set or in some alternating fashion with the full range reps. For example, after performing a set of *biceps curls* to failure, an individual would cheat the bar back to the most contracted position, and then perform several partial reps.

Other Techniques

Progressive movement training

Progressive movement training attempts to gradually increase the range of motion throughout a training cycle. The lifter will start with a much heavier weight than they could handle in the full range of motion, only moving through the last 3–5" of the movement. Throughout the training cycle, the lifter will gradually increase the range of motion until the joint moves through the full range of the exercise. This is a style that was made popular by Paul Anderson.

Super slow

Super slow repetitions are performed with lighter weights. The lifting and lowering phases of each repetition take 10 seconds or more.

Timed rests

By strictly controlling the rest periods between reps and sets a trainer can reduce their level of blood oxygenation, which helps to increase the stress on the muscles.

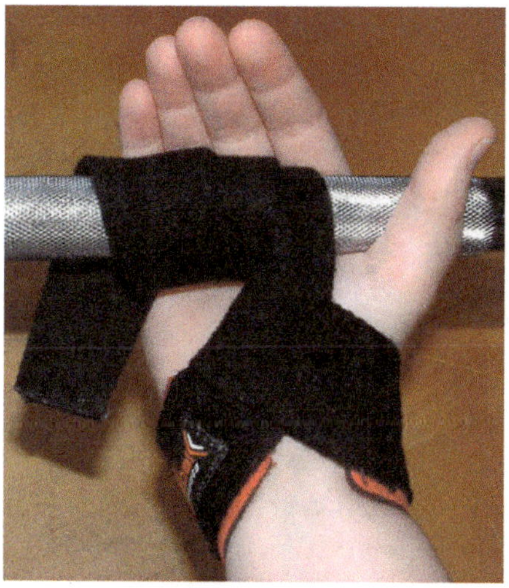

Using a wrist strap

Wrist straps

Wrist straps (lifting straps) are sometimes used to assist in gripping very heavy weights. Wrist straps can be used to isolate muscle groups like in "lat pull-downs", where the trainee would primarily use the latissimus dorsi muscles of the back rather than the biceps. They are particularly useful for the *deadlift*. Some lifters avoid using wrist straps to develop their grip strength, just as some go further by using thick bars. Wrist straps can allow a lifter initially to use more weight than they might be able to handle safely for an entire set, as unlike simply holding a weight, if it is dropped then the lifter must descend with it or be pulled down. Straps place stress on the bones of the wrist which can be potentially harmful if excessive.

Risks and Concerns

Strength training is a safe form of exercise when the movements are controlled, and carefully defined. Or some safety measures can also be taken before the training. However, as with any form of exercise, improper execution and the failure to take appropriate precautions can result in injury. A helmet, boots, gloves, and back belt can aide in injury prevention. Principles of weight training safety apply to strength training.

Bodybuilding

Bodybuilding is a sport in which the goal is to increase muscle size and definition. Bodybuilding increases the endurance of muscles, as well as strength, though not as much as if it were the primary goal. Bodybuilders compete in bodybuilding competitions, and use specific principles and methods of strength training to maximize muscular size and develop extremely low levels of body fat. In contrast, most strength trainers train to improve their strength and endurance while not giving special attention to reducing body fat below normal. Strength trainers tend to focus on compound exercises to build basic strength, whereas bodybuilders often use isolation exercises to visually separate their muscles, and to improve muscular symmetry. Pre-contest training for bodybuilders is different again, in that they attempt to retain as much muscular tissue as possible while undergoing severe dieting. However, the bodybuilding community has been the source of many strength training principles, techniques, vocabulary, and customs.

Nutrition

It is widely accepted that strength training must be matched by changes in diet in order to be effective. Although aerobic exercise has been proven to have an effect on the dietary intake of macronutrients, strength training has not and an increase in dietary protein is generally believed to be required for building skeletal muscle with popular sources advising weight trainers to consume a high-protein diet which delivers 1.4 to 1.8 g of protein per kg of body weight per day (0.6 to 0.8 g per pound). Protein that is neither needed for cell growth and repair nor consumed for energy is converted into urea mainly through the deamination process and is excreted by the kidneys. It was once thought that a high-protein diet entails risk of kidney damage, but studies have shown that kidney problems only occur in people with previous kidney disease. However failure to properly hydrate can put an increased strain on the kidney's ability to function. An adequate supply of carbohydrates (5–7 g per kg) is also needed as a source of energy and for the body to restore glycogen levels in muscles.

A light, balanced meal prior to the workout (usually one to two hours beforehand) ensures that adequate energy and amino acids are available for the intense bout of exercise. The type of nutrients consumed affects the response of the body, and nutrient timing whereby protein and carbohydrates are consumed prior to and after workout has a beneficial impact on muscle growth. Water is consumed throughout the course of the workout to prevent poor performance due to dehydration. A protein shake is often consumed immediately following the workout, because both protein uptake and protein usage are increased at this time. Glucose (or another simple sugar) is often consumed as well since this quickly replenishes any glycogen lost during the exercise period. To maximise muscle protein anabolism, recovery drink should contain glucose (dextrose), protein (usually whey) hydrolysate containing mainly dipeptides and tripeptides, and leucine. Some weight trainers also take ergogenic aids such as creatine or steroids to aid muscle growth. However, the effectiveness of some products is disputed and others are potentially harmful.

Sex Differences in Mass Gains

Due to the androgenic hormonal differences between males and females, the latter are generally unable to develop large muscles regardless of the training program used. Normally the most that can be achieved is a look similar to that of a fitness model. Muscle is denser than fat, so someone who builds muscle while keeping the same body weight will occupy less volume; if two people weigh the same (and are the same height) but have different lean body mass percentages, the one with more muscle will appear thinner.

In addition, though bodybuilding uses the same principles as strength training, it is with a goal of gaining muscle bulk. Strength trainers with different goals and programs will not gain the same mass as a professional bodybuilder.

Muscle Toning

Some weight trainers perform light, high-repetition exercises in an attempt to "tone" their muscles without increasing their size.

The word tone derives from the Latin "tonus" (meaning "tension"). In anatomy and physiology, as well as medicine, the term "muscle tone" refers to the continuous and passive partial contraction of the muscles, or the muscles' resistance to passive stretching during resting state as determined by a deep tendon reflex. Muscle tonus is dependent on neurological input into the muscle. In medicine, observations of changes in muscle tonus can be used to determine normal or abnormal states which can be indicative of pathology. The common strength training term "tone" is derived from this use.

What muscle builders refer to as a *toned physique* or "muscle firmness" is one that combines reasonable muscular size with moderate levels of body fat, qualities that may result from a combination of diet and exercise.

Muscle tone or firmness is derived from the increase in actin and myosin cross filaments in the sarcomere. When this occurs the same amount of neurological input creates a greater firmness or tone in the resting continuous and passive partial contraction in the muscle.

Exercises of 6–12 reps cause hypertrophy of the sarcoplasm in slow-twitch and high-twitch muscle fibers, contributing to overall increased muscle bulk. It is different from myofibril hypertrophy which leads to strength gains. Both however can occur to an extent during this rep range. *Even though most are of the opinion that higher repetitions are best for producing the desired effect of muscle firmness or tone, it is not.* Low volume strength training of 5 repetitions or fewer will increase strength by increasing actin and myosin cross filaments thereby increasing muscle firmness or tone. The low volume of this training will inhibit the hypertrophy effect.

Lowered-calorie diets have no positive effect on muscle hypertrophy for muscle of any fiber type. They may, however, decrease the thickness of subcutaneous fat (fat between muscle and skin), through an overall reduction in body fat, thus making muscle striations more visible.

Weight Loss

Exercises like sit-ups, or abdominal crunches, performs less work than whole-body aerobic exercises thereby expending fewer calories during exercise than jogging, for example.

Hypertrophy serves to maintain muscle mass, for an elevated basal metabolic rate, which has the potential to burn more calories in a given period compared to aerobics. This helps to maintain a higher metabolic rate which would otherwise diminish after metabolic adaption to dieting, or upon completion of an aerobic routine.

Weight loss also depends on the type of strength training used. Weight training is generally used for bulking, but the bulking method will more than likely not increase weight because of the diet involved. However, when resistance or circuit training is used, because they are not geared towards bulking, women tend to lose weight more quickly. Lean muscles require calories to maintain themselves at rest, which will help reduce fat through an increase in the basal metabolic rate.

History

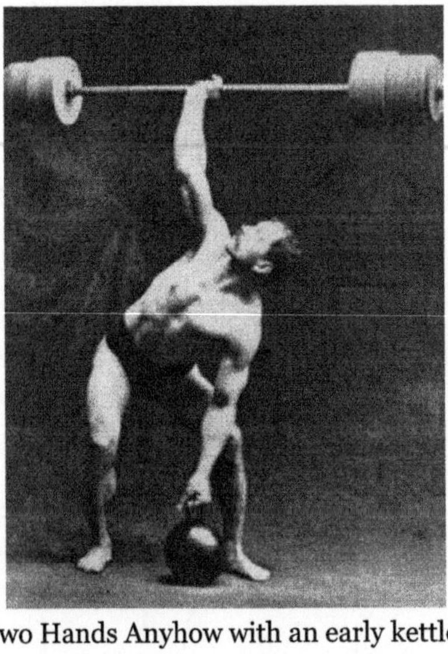

Arthur Saxon performing a Two Hands Anyhow with an early kettlebell and plate-loaded barbell

Until the 20th century, the history of strength training was very similar to the history of weight training. With the advent of modern technology, materials and knowledge, the methods that can be used for strength training have multiplied significantly.

Hippocrates explained the principle behind strength training when he wrote "that which is used develops, and that which is not used wastes away", referring to muscular hypertrophy and atrophy. Progressive resistance training dates back at least to Ancient Greece, when legend has it that wrestler Milo of Croton trained by carrying a newborn calf on his back every day until it was fully grown. Another Greek, the physician Galen, described strength training exercises using the halteres (an early form of dumbbell) in the 2nd century. Ancient Persians used the *meels*, which became popular during the 19th century as the Indian club, and has recently made a comeback in the form of the clubbell.

The dumbbell was joined by the barbell in the latter half of the 19th century. Early barbells had hollow globes that could be filled with sand or lead shot, but by the end of the century these were replaced by the plate-loading barbell commonly used today.

Strength training with isometric exercise was popularised by Charles Atlas from the 1930s onwards. The 1960s saw the gradual introduction of exercise machines into the still-rare strength training gyms of the time. Strength training became increasingly popular in the 1980s following the release of the bodybuilding movie *Pumping Iron* and the subsequent popularity of Arnold Schwarzenegger.

Special Populations

Safety Concerns Related to Children

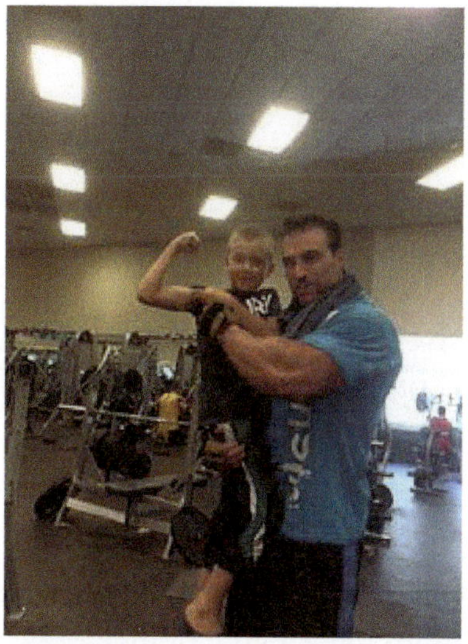

Properly supervised strength training for children

Orthopaedic specialists used to recommend that children avoid weight training because the growth plates on their bones might be at risk. The very rare reports of growth plate fractures in children who trained with weights occurred as a result of inadequate supervision, improper form or excess weight, and there have been no reports of injuries to growth plates in youth training programs that followed established guidelines. The position of the National Strength and Conditioning Association is that strength training is safe for children if properly designed and supervised.

Younger children are at greater risk of injury than adults if they drop a weight on themselves or perform an exercise incorrectly; further, they may lack understanding of, or ignore the safety precautions around weight training equipment. As a result, supervision of minors is considered vital to ensuring the safety of any youth engaging in strength training.

Australia's Stance on Pre-adolescence Strength Training

Strength training is the fourth most popular form of fitness in Australia. Due to its popularity amongst all ages, there is great scepticism on what the appropriate age to commence strength training in young athletes is. Some points of the opposing view of strength training in young adolescence are stunted growth, health and bone problems in later stages of life and unhealthy eating habits. Studies by Australian experts that have been recognised by the Australian Institute of Sport (AIS) have debunked these myths. There is no link between any prolonged health risks and strength training in pre-adolescence if the procedures of strength training are followed correctly and under suitable supervision. Strength training for pre-adolescents should focus on skills and techniques. Children should only work on strengthening all the big muscle groups, using free weight and body weight movements with relatively light loads. The benefits of these practices include increased strength performance, injury prevention and learning good training principles.

For Older Adults

Older adults are prone to loss of muscle strength. With more strength older adults have better health, better quality of life, better physical function and fewer falls. In cases in which an older person begins strength training, their doctor or health care provider may neglect to emphasize a strength training program which results in muscle gains. Under-dosed strength training programs should be avoided in favor of a program which matches the abilities and goals of the person exercising.

In setting up an exercise program for an older adult, they should go through a baseline fitness assessment to determine their current limits. Any exercise program for older adults should match the intensity, frequency, and duration of exercise that the person can perform. The program should have a goal of increased strength as compared to the baseline measurement.

Recommended training for older adults is three times a week of light strength training exercises. Exercise machines are a commonly used equipment in a gym setting, including treadmills with exercises such as walking or light jogging. Home-based exercises should usually consist of body weight or elastic band exercises that maintain a low level of impact on the muscles. Weights can also be used by older adults if they maintain a lighter weight load with an average amount of repetitions (10–12 REPS) with suitable supervision. It is important for older adults to maintain a light level of strength training with low levels of impact to avoid injuries.

Older people who exercise against a resistance or force become stronger . Progressive resistance training (PRT) also improves physical functioning in older people, including the performance of simple (e.g.: walking, climbing stairs, rising from a chair more quickly) and complex daily activities (e.g.: bathing, cooking). Caution is recommended when transferring PRT exercises for clinical populations,as adverse effects are unclear.

Eccentric Training

An eccentric contraction is the motion of an active muscle while it is lengthening under load. Eccentric training is repetitively doing eccentric muscle contractions. For example, in a biceps curl the action of lowering the dumbbell back down from the lift is the eccentric phase of that exercise — as long as the dumbbell is lowered slowly rather than letting it drop (i.e., the biceps are in a state of contraction to control the rate of descent of the dumbbell).

An eccentric contraction is one of the three distinct phases in the movement of muscles and tendons, the other two are an isometric contraction (no movement), and a concentric contraction (contracting).

Eccentric training focuses on slowing down the elongation of the muscle process in order to challenge the muscles, which can lead to stronger muscles, faster muscle repair and increasing metabolic rate.

Eccentric movement provides a braking mechanism for muscle and tendon groups that are experiencing concentric movement to protect joints from damage as the contraction is released.

Eccentric training is particularly good for casual and high performance athletes or the elderly and patients looking to rehabilitate certain muscles and tendons.

Negative Movement

This movement has also been described as negative training. This "negative" movement is necessary to reverse the muscle from its initial trajectory.

When weight exceeds the force developed by the muscle, as in an eccentric muscle action, the exercise is referred to as negative work because the muscle is absorbing energy in this loaded position.

Eccentric contractions use less energy, even though they create more force than concentric actions.

History

Adolf Fick originally discovered in 1882 that "contracting muscle under stretch could produce greater force than a shortening muscle contraction" like in concentric movements. Fifty years later, A.V. Hill determined that "the body had lower energy demand during an eccentric muscle contraction than during a concentric muscle action".

Erling Asmussen first introduced eccentric training in 1953 as "excentric," with ex meaning "away from" and centric meaning "center." Hence, the term was coined to mean a muscle contraction that moves away from the center of the muscle.

But the first revelation of the functional significance of these properties occurred by way of a clever demonstration devised by Bud Abbott, Brenda Bigland, and Murdoch Ritchie. They connected two stationary cycle ergometers back-to-back with a single chain, such that one cyclist pedaled forward and the other resisted this forward motion by braking the backward-moving pedals. Because the internal resistance of the device was low, the same force was being applied by both individuals, yet the task was much easier for the individual braking. This demonstration cleverly revealed that a tiny female resisting the movement of the pedals could easily exert more force than, and hence control the power output of, a large burly male pedaling forward.

Energy

During the eccentric phase of movement, the muscle absorbs energy. This work is done "by stretching the muscle and in this process the muscle absorbs mechanical energy".

This mechanical energy is dissipated or converted into one or a combination of two energies.

- Heat
- Elastic recoil

Heat

The energy that is absorbed by the muscle will be dissipated as heat if the muscle is being used as a "damper or shock absorber". This leads to increase in body temperature.

Elastic Recoil

The energy that is absorbed by the muscle can be converted into elastic recoil energy, and can be recovered and reused by the body. This creates more efficiency because the body is able to use the energy for the next movement, decreasing the initial impact or shock of the movement.

For example, kinetic energy is absorbed in running every time one's foot strikes the ground and continues as one's mass overtakes the foot. At this moment, elastic recoil energy is at its maximum and a large amount of this energy is absorbed and is added to the next stride.

This movement is similar to the action of springs, where the muscle is continually shortened and stretched resulting in enhanced effectiveness and force. It can lead to the perception of "less effort" even though dealing with higher force.

But time matters in elastic recoil. If this energy is not used quickly it is dissipated as heat. The role of eccentric training is to use these principles of energy conversion to strengthen muscle and tendon groups.

Physiological Mechanisms

The muscle has "tension producing tissue comprising small contractile units referred to as sarcomeres" that each contain a "thick (myosin) and thin (actin) myofilament (muscle filaments or proteins) that overlaps to format a cross-bridge bond (attachment)".

When in a concentric exercise, shortening of a muscle occurs as the myosin and actin cross bridges repeatedly attach and detach to draw the actin across the myosin – creating force. Each cross-bridge attachment and detachment cycle is powered by the splitting of one molecule of adenosine triphosphate (ATP). Examples of such exercises include kicking a ball or lifting a weight.

In controlled release reversals of such concentric motions, the eccentric movement stretches the muscle with opposing force that is stronger than the muscle force. When myofilaments of the muscle fiber are stretched in such eccentric contractions there can be reduced numbers of detachments of cross bridge myosin and actin links. With more cross bridges remaining attached there is greater force production in the muscle. Examples of activities involving eccentric muscle contraction include walking down a hill or resisting the force of gravity while lowering a heavy object.

"Eccentric actions place a stretch on the sarcomeres to the point where the myofilaments may experience strain, otherwise known as exercise induced delayed onset muscle soreness (DOMS)" (Aaron Bubbico & Len Kravitz, 2010). One area of research that has much promise in relation to DOMS and eccentric exercise is the repeated-bout effect (RBE). To help prevent or lessen DOMS from eccentric exercise, or to facilitate recovery from it, the exerciser would eccentrically stimulate the muscle then repeat at weekly intervals to build up strength and allow the strain (in response to a given force level) to reduce over time.

Muscle Injury

Eccentric contractions are a frequent cause of muscle injury when engaging in unaccustomed exercise. But a single bout of such eccentric exercise leads to adaptation which will make the muscle less vulnerable to injury on subsequent performance of the eccentric exercise.

Findings

Several key findings have been researched regarding the benefits of eccentric training:

- Eccentric training creates greater force owing to the "decreased rate of cross-bridge muscle detachments." Patients and athletes will have more muscle force for bigger weights when eccentric training.
- Eccentric contractions use less energy and actually absorb energy that will be used as heat or elastic recoil for the next movement.
- Increased DOMS leads to more tenderness in eccentric, rather than pure pain or tendon swelling amongst patients.
- Repeated-bout Effect markedly reduces DOMS. "Completing bouts of eccentric training and then repeating the workout 1 week (or more) later will result in less DOMS after the second workout."
- Older individuals are less vulnerable to injury from eccentric exercise, primarily because of the reduced strain on muscle-tendon groupings as compared to traditional concentric exercise.
- Stretching of the muscles and eccentric training provides protection from injury or re-injury.
- Eccentric training has proven to be an excellent post rehabilitation intervention for lower-body injuries.
- Subjects report less weariness from eccentric training than from concentric training.
- Total body eccentric training can raise resting metabolic rate by about 9 percent, with the greatest magnitude in the first two hours.
- While energy costs remain low, the degree of force is very high. This leads to muscles that respond with significant increases in muscle strength, size and power.

Eccentric Exercise

Eccentric exercise or resistance training is currently being used as a form of rehabilitation for sport injuries, but also as an alternative form of exercise for the elderly, those affected by neurological disorders, COPD, cardiopulmonary disorders, and cancer. Muscle loss is a big problem faced by the people afflicted with the above disorders and many cannot participate in rigorous exercise protocols. Eccentric muscle contractions produce high forces with low-energy cost. According to Hortobágyi due to these properties eccentric exercise has the greatest potential for muscle strengthening. To strengthen muscle the external force must exceed the muscle while it lengthens. The definition of eccentric contraction is almost the exact definition of muscle strengthening.

1. Perceived Muscle Damage: There is a stipulation regarding eccentric contractions in that they actually cause muscle damage and injury. Eccentric contraction may result in delayed onset muscle soreness however; the contraction itself does not cause muscle damage or injury.

2. Proof of Muscle Strengthening w/o Damage: One recurring problem in ACL rehabilitation is improving muscle strength of the quadriceps without re-injury. Early, high-force eccentric training can be used to increase muscle strength and volume without damage to the ACL graft, surrounding soft-tissue, and the articular cartilage. In an experiment performed on rat muscles after twenty sessions of treadmill low intensity eccentric training the wet weight of the muscles and the fiber cross-section were significantly larger than the control and level groups. These results led to the conclusion that low intensity eccentric contractions have the ability to "produce enough mechanical stress to induce muscle hypertrophy without over-stressing which could produce muscle fiber damage. Other articles have found that muscle damage is not required to reach hypertrophy. Greater mechanical stress brought on by eccentric contractions is what leads to hypertrophy in individuals undergoing eccentric training. Studies done on the elderly show that low-intensity eccentric conditioning can actually minimize muscle damage According to Gault the low cost of energy, and low oxygen demand make low-intensity eccentric exercise ideal for the elderly.

3. Eccentric Contraction and Oxygen Consumption: Oxygen consumption is needed for muscles to work properly. Eccentric muscle contractions are considered to be negative work as the muscle is working with resistance. Negative work is the mechanical energy absorbed by the work conducted on a muscle when the force on the muscle is greater than the force produced. An experiment was conducted on bicycle riding. The amount of oxygen consumption was measured during the motion of pedaling forward as positive work and pedaling with resistance as negative work. Less oxygen was consumed during negative work then that of positive work with the oxygen consumption ratio being 3:7. Due to the low oxygen consumption of eccentric exercise studies have been conducted on patients with severe COPD. An eccentric cycling exercise workout was created for these patients and the results found there to be no side effects, minimal muscle soreness that had no effect on power, and a high compliance. Further-

more, other cycling studies concluded that eccentric cycling was a safe alternative for COPD patients as they can perform high intensity work with lower cost.

4. Eccentric Contractions and Cardiac Output: With lower cost of oxygen how would eccentric exercise affect the heart? A study was performed to test how eccentric and concentric contractions effect cardiac autonomic modulation after exercise. Men (aged 18–30) were divided into four groups: concentric control, eccentric control, concentric training, and eccentric training. Results concluded that resistance training (eccentric contractions) promoted strength gain. An increase in cardiac vagal modulation during recovery was also concluded.

A lot of studies have been conducted regarding eccentric exercise over the last decade. It can be said there is substantial evidence that eccentric exercise truly exceeds concentric exercise for rehabilitation and training aspects in force, energy cost, oxygen consumption, and muscular strengthening.

Sports and Rehabilitation

With eccentric training, muscles are able to create more for less work, which has special meaning in the realms of high performance sports — both for injury prevention and optimal-performance training. For athletes and sports enthusiasts, this eccentric model can help with explosive force training in order to prevent injuries or recurring injuries, and trains the body to use the kinetic force driven by eccentric training more efficiently. Canadian Olympian Kim St. Pierre uses eccentric training as part of her regime. The Esmonde Technique takes eccentric training and makes it available to the masses through Classical Stretch and Essentrics. After having hip surgery in the summer of 2007, St.Pierre began to practice the Esmonde Technique with experts Miranda Esmonde-White from PBS's Classical Stretch and Sahra Esmonde-White host of the Essentrics workout in order to heal her hip.

According to tests, increases in both strength and muscle fiber are higher in eccentric training than in traditional concentric training.

The rehabilitative nature, low energy costs, high magnitudes of force, and low uptake of oxygen all align eccentric exercise for both the elderly and rehabilitative functions.

In old age, loss of strength and muscle mass is commonplace. Add to these factors disease and cardiac and respiratory illness. Eccentric training enables the elderly, and those with the same problems, the ability to train muscle groups and increase strength and resiliency with low-energy exercise.

Eccentric training has been found to be beneficial to those with a variety of physical ailments.

Anterior Cruciate Ligament (ACL) Damage

Tearing an ACL in the knee causes serious damage that can last several years and often requires surgery. The ACL is one of the four main stabilizing ligaments of the knee. During the post-operative rehabilitation of patients, eccentric training can be used as a cornerstone of developing muscle size and strength. According to tests conducted J. Parry Gerber in 2007, structural changes in the muscles greatly exceeded those achieved with standard concentric rehabilitation. The success of the involvement of gradual progressive exposure to negative work ultimately led to the production of high muscle force.

Sarcopenia

Sarcopenia is the progressive loss of muscle mass due to aging. Muscle mass begins to deteriorate as early as the age of 25, and consistently deteriorates into old age. By the age of 80 "one half of the skeletal muscle has been lost" (Lastayo, Woolf, Lewek, Snyder-Mackler, Reich & Lindstedt, 2003). With this great decrease in mass, strength is also decreased. Eccentric training has the ability to counteract sarcopenia through sustained training. The unique trait of greater overloads to the muscle with less strenuous impact on the body, as well as cardiac and respiratory systems, offers a unique case for the elderly. The high-force and low-cost set of attributes in eccentric exercise makes it ideal for the actively impaired.

Muscle Tendon Injuries

The entire muscle-tendon system works cohesively to slow down limb movement. The close relationship between the muscle and tendons help to dissipate heat or temporarily store kinetic energy. If the forces needed to slow down a limb exceed the capacity of the muscle-tendon system, injury is likely to occur.

Athletes with recurring hamstring and abductor muscle injuries have greater impairment of eccentric strength, suggesting that improvements in eccentric training may minimize the risks of injury by strengthening the muscle-tendon groupings in high-stress areas of the body.

Eccentric training is of huge benefit to those that wish to avert injuries by improving the muscles abilities to absorb more energy before deteriorating. According to one article, "Increased stiffness in tendons, greater force at failure, and an improved ability to absorb energy at the musculotendonous junction result following eccentric exercise training".

Osteopenia

Usually viewed as a precursor to osteoporosis, osteopenia is when bone density is lower than normal levels. Bone mass is affected by muscles forces and their loads to the bone structure. The strength and density of the bone is directly influenced by local strain.

Due to the high strain on muscles during eccentric training, coupled with low energy output, eccentric training becomes a cornerstone of the rehabilitative process.

Tendinoses

Intense repetitive activities tend to create chronic tendon disorders, where the tendons become injured, inflamed or ruptured. While typically these disorders are directly related to eccentric muscle movements, the ability for a muscle to strengthen and prevent injury through eccentric training is great. Controlled rehabilitative regimes will actually strengthen and repair tendons. Ample evidence supports the notion that the tendon, like the muscle, can adapt favorably to physical stress and eccentric loads.

It has been deduced that high muscle tendon forces delivered in a controlled environment are needed for optimal tendon adaptation. While eccentric stress is related to the injury, high force eccentric exercises are needed to maximize recovery.

Chronic Patellar Tendonitis

A condition that arises when the tendon and the tissues that surround it, become inflamed and irritated. This is usually due to overuse, especially from jumping activities. This is the reason chronic patellar tendonitis is often called "jumper's knee." A study done by Roald Bahr and colleagues looked at which method of tendon rehabilitation exercise — the "eccentric squat" exercise or the universal gym "leg extension/leg curl" — produced more recovery results in terms of recovery in the treatment of chronic patellar tendonitis. On the twelve-week exercise program, participants were tested for thigh circumference and quadriceps and hamstring moment of force. There was no significant difference between the groups in either quadriceps or hamstring moment of force and hamstring moment of force significantly increased in both groups, but the eccentric squat saw significantly lower pain ratings and produced twice as many "pain free" subjects at the end of the program than the other group.

Suspension Training

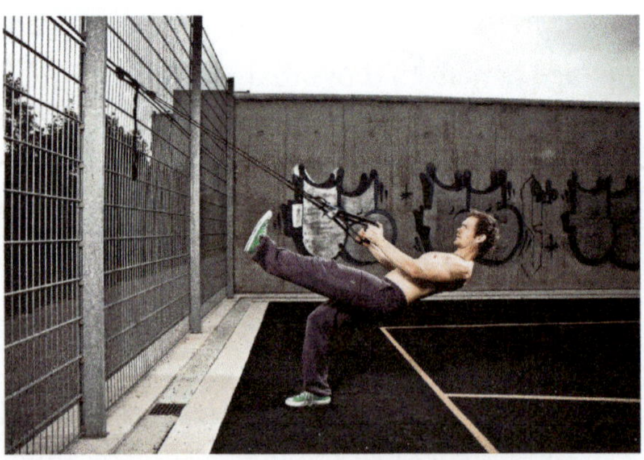

outdoor workout with a Sling Trainer

The term suspension training refers to an approach to strength training that uses a system of ropes and webbing called a "suspension trainer" to allow users to work against their own body weight.

Description

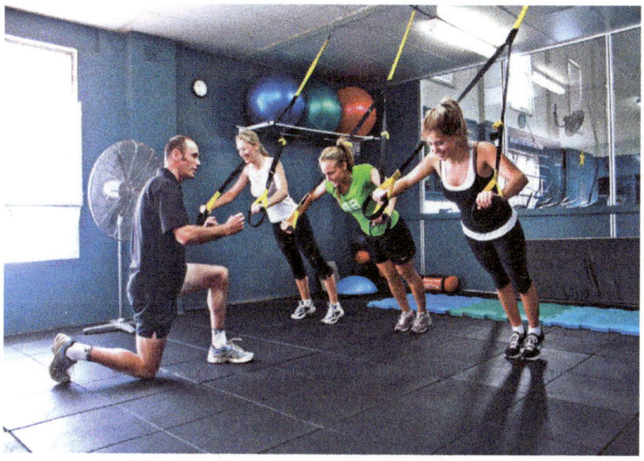

Group suspension training

The field of suspension training is a form of resistance training that includes body-weight exercises in which a variety of multi-planar, compound exercise movements can be performed. These are done with the aim of developing strength, balance, flexibility, and joint stability simultaneously. Suspension training develops physical strength while using functional movements and dynamic positions. The actual term "suspension training" is a trademark of FITNESS ANYWHERE, LLC.

History

Rope training has been around as early as the 1800s.

Randy Hetrick, a former Navy Seal and Stanford MBA graduate, developed the Total Resistance eXercise (TRX) equipment and the associated Suspension Training body-weight exercises in the 1990s, and started marketing it in 2005. Kurt Dasbach, a former professional soccer player in Chile, discovered an ancient Andean conditioning system that utilized ropes while playing in South America and developed a rival product, Inkaflexx, around the same time. Inkaflexx has since closed shop, but TRX continues as a $60 million per year business.

In 2008, ex Bristol City F.C. fitness coaching team Mark Hammond and Pete Faulkner developed the FKPro two-strap system. In 2009 Fabio Martella MMA coaching wrote the first TRX technical manual in Italy. Another alternative is the aeroSling ELITE made in Germany. This "Suspended Pulley Trainer" also contains a pulley system. The Hook Isometrics/Suspension Trainer by Sierra Exercise Equipment enables the user to use it for either suspension training or isometrics training. Evolution has continued with TRX and other companies improving designs to minimize risk.

Benefits and Criticism

Proponents of suspension training argue that it develops core body strength, as well as joint and muscular stability, reducing the chance of injury. Some sports scientists have expressed concern that weaker individuals may not have the core stability or joint integrity to use the system safely and effectively.

Circuit Training

Circuit training is a form of body conditioning or resistance training using high-intensity aerobics. It targets strength building or muscular endurance. An exercise "circuit" is one completion of all prescribed exercises in the program. When one circuit is complete, one begins the first exercise again for the next circuit. Traditionally, the time between exercises in circuit training is short, often with rapid movement to the next exercise.

The program was developed by R.E. Morgan and G.T. Adamson in 1957 at the University of Leeds in England.

Typical Activities in a Circuit Training

A circuit should work each section of the body individually. Typical activities include:

Upper-body

- Squat ups
- Bench dips
- Back extensions
- Medicine ball chest pass
- Bench lift
- Inclined press up

Core & Trunk

- Sit ups (lower abdominal)
- Stomach crunch (upper abdominal)
- Back extension chest raise

Lower-body

- Squat jumps
- Compass jumps

- Astride jumps
- Step ups
- Shuttle runs
- Hopping shuttles
- Bench squat

Total-body

- Burpees
- Treadmills
- Squat thrusts
- Skipping
- Jogging

Effects of Circuit Training

Studies at Baylor University and The Cooper Institute show that circuit training is the most time efficient way to enhance cardiovascular fitness and muscle endurance. Studies show that circuit training helps women to achieve their goals and maintain them longer than other forms of exercise or diet.

Morgan and Anderson claim:

> "Perhaps a most profound finding of this study, from a health perspective, is that this investigation clearly shows that performance of this circuit of exercises,this level of intensity elicited oxygen consumption values (39% to 51.5% of VO2max) that meet established guidelines of the American College of Sports Medicine (ACSM) for the recommended intensity (40% to 85% of VO2maxR) of exercise for developing and maintaining cardio-respiratory fitness. Thus, this circuit not only provides a suitable muscular fitness stimulus but also helps to meet ACSM cardiovascular guidelines and the newly published Dietary Guidelines for Americans 2005 for physical activity."

One advantage is that reduced station times will encourage the participants to lift heavier weights, which means they can achieve overload with smaller number of repetitions: typically in the range of 25 to 50 depending on their training goals.

Weight Training

Weight training is a common type of strength training for developing the strength and size of skeletal muscles. It utilizes the force of gravity in the form of weighted bars, dumbbells or weight stacks in order to oppose the force generated by muscle through concentric or eccentric contraction. Weight training uses a variety of specialized equipment to target specific muscle groups and types of movement.

Sports where strength training is central are bodybuilding, weightlifting, powerlifting, and strongman, highland games, shot put, discus throw, and javelin throw. Many other sports use strength training as part of their training regimen, notably; mixed martial arts, American football, wrestling, rugby football, track and field, rowing, lacrosse, basketball, baseball, and hockey. Strength training for other sports and physical activities is becoming increasingly popular.

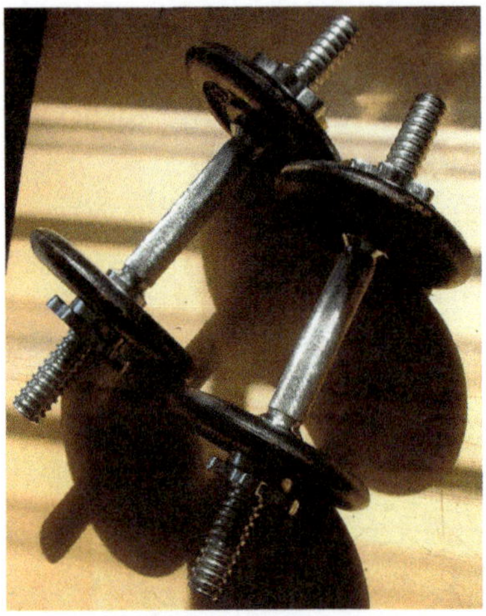

A complete weight training workout can be performed with a pair of adjustable dumbbells and a set of weight disks (plates)

Weight Training Versus Other Types of Exercise

Strength training is an inclusive term that describes all exercises devoted toward increasing physical strength. Weight training is a type of strength training that uses weights, Eccentric Training or muscular resistance to increase strength. Endurance training is associated with aerobic exercise while flexibility training is associated with stretching exercise like yoga or pilates. *Weight training* is often used as a synonym for strength training, but is actually a specific type within the more inclusive category. Contrary to popular belief, weight training can be beneficial for both men and women.

History

The genealogy of lifting can be traced back to the beginning of history where humanity's fascination with physical abilities can be found among numerous ancient writings. Progressive resistance training dates back at least to Ancient Greece, when legend has it that wrestler Milo of Croton trained by carrying a newborn calf on his back every day until it was fully grown. Another Greek, the physician Galen, described strength training exercises using the halteres (an early form of dumbbell) in the 2nd century.

Ancient Greek sculptures also depict lifting feats. The weights were generally stones, but later gave way to dumbbells. The dumbbell was joined by the barbell in the later half of the 19th century. Early barbells had hollow globes that could be filled with sand or lead shot, but by the end of the century these were replaced by the plate-loading barbell commonly used today.

Another early device was the Indian club, which came from ancient Persia where it was called the "meels". It subsequently became popular during the 19th century, and has recently made a comeback in the form of the clubbell.

The 1960s saw the gradual introduction of exercise machines into the still-rare strength training gyms of the time. Weight training became increasingly popular in the 1970s, following the release of the bodybuilding movie *Pumping Iron,* and the subsequent popularity of Arnold Schwarzenegger. Since the late 1990s increasing numbers of women have taken up weight training, influenced by programs like Body for Life; currently nearly one in five U.S. women engage in weight training on a regular basis.

Basic Principles

The basic principles of weight training are essentially identical to those of strength training, and involve a manipulation of the number of repetitions (reps), sets, tempo, exercise types, and weight moved to cause desired increases in strength, endurance, and size. The specific combinations of reps, sets, exercises, and weights depends on the aims of the individual performing the exercise. Sets with fewer reps can be performed with heavier weights contributing to an increase in lean muscle mass and sets with higher reps can be performed with lighter weights contributing to increased muscular endurance.

In addition to the basic principles of *strength training,* a further consideration added by weight training is the equipment used. Types of equipment include barbells, dumbbells, pulleys and stacks in the form of weight machines, and the body's own weight in the case of chin-ups and push-ups. Different types of weights will give different types of resistance, and often the same absolute weight can have different relative weights depending on the type of equipment used. For example, lifting 10 kilograms using a dumbbell sometimes requires more force than moving 10 kilograms on a weight stack if certain pulley arrangements are used. In other cases, the weight stack may require more force than the equivalent dumbbell weight due to additional torque or resistance in the machine. Additionally, although they may display the same weight stack, different machines may be heavier or lighter depending on the number of pulleys and their arrangements.

Weight training also requires the use of 'good form', performing the movements with the appropriate muscle group, and not transferring the weight to different body parts in order to move greater weight (called 'cheating'). Failure to use good form during a training set can result in injury or a failure to meet training goals; since the desired muscle group is not challenged sufficiently, the threshold of overload is never reached and the muscle does not gain in strength. At a particularly advanced level; however, "cheating" can be used to break through strength plateaus and encourage neurological and muscular adaptation.

Comparison to Other Types of Strength Training

The benefits of weight training overall are comparable to most other types of strength training: increased muscle, tendon and ligament strength, bone density, flexibility, tone, metabolic rate, and postural support. This type of training will also help prevent injury for athletes. There are benefits and limitations to weight training as compared to other types of strength training.

Weight Training Versus Isometric Training

Isometric exercise provides a maximum amount of resistance based on the force output of the muscle, or muscles pitted against one another. This maximum force maximally strengthens the muscles over all of the joint angles at which the isometric exercise occurs. By comparison, weight training also strengthens the muscle throughout the range of motion the joint is trained in, but only maximally at one angle, causing a lesser increase in physical strength at other angles from the initial through terminating joint angle as compared with isometric exercise. In addition, the risk of injury from weights used in weight training is greater than with isometric exercise (no weights), and the risk of asymmetric training is also greater than with isometric exercise of identical opposing muscles.

Weight Training and Bodybuilding

Although weight training is similar to bodybuilding, they have different objectives. Bodybuilders use weight training to develop their muscles for size, shape, and symmetry regardless of any increase in strength for competition in bodybuilding contests; they train to maximize their muscular size and develop extremely low levels of body fat. In contrast, many weight trainers train to improve their strength and anaerobic endurance while not giving special attention to reducing body fat far below normal.

The bodybuilding community has been the source of many of weight training's principles, techniques, vocabulary, and customs. Weight training does allow tremendous flexibility in exercises and weights which can allow bodybuilders to target specific muscles and muscle groups, as well as attain specific goals. Not all bodybuilding is undertaken to compete in bodybuilding contests and, in fact, the vast majority of bodybuilders never compete, but bodybuild for their own personal reasons.

Safety

Weight training is a safe form of exercise when the movements are controlled and carefully defined. However, as with any form of exercise, improper execution and the failure to take appropriate precautions can result in injury.

Maintaining Proper Form

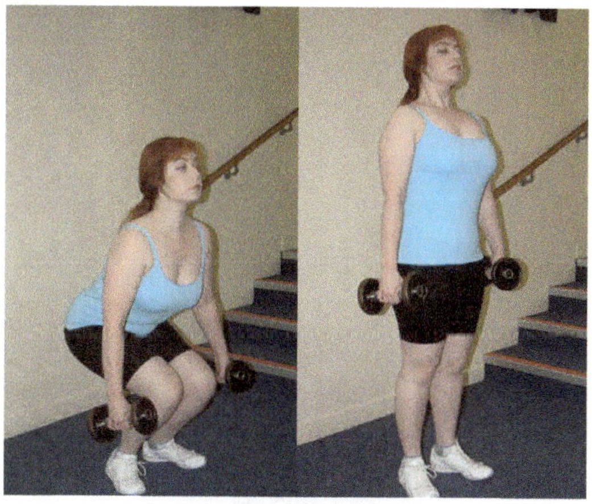

A dumbbell half-squat

Maintaining proper form is one of the many steps in order to perfectly perform a certain technique. Correct form in weight training improves strength, muscle tone, and maintaining a healthy weight. Proper form will prevent any strains or fractures. When the exercise becomes difficult towards the end of a set, there is a temptation to cheat, i.e., to use poor form to recruit other muscle groups to assist the effort. Avoid heavy weight and keep the number of repetitions to a minimum. This may shift the effort to weaker muscles that cannot handle the weight. For example, the *squat* and the *deadlift* are used to exercise the largest muscles in the body—the leg and buttock muscles—so they require substantial weight. Beginners are tempted to round their back while performing these exercises. The relaxation of the spinal erectors which allows the lower back to round can cause shearing in the vertebrae of the lumbar spine, potentially damaging the spinal discs.

Stretching and Warm-up

Weight trainers commonly spend 5 to 20 minutes warming up their muscles before starting a workout. It is common to stretch the entire body to increase overall flexibility; however, many people stretch just the area being worked that day. The main reason for warming up is injury prevention. Warming up increases blood flow and flexibility, which lessens the chance of a muscle pull or joint pain.

Warm up sets are also important. For example, the same lifter working on his chest would also be advised to complete at least two warm up sets prior to hitting his "core tonnage." Core tonnage refers to the heavier lifts that actually strain your muscles. For example, if the lifter's main sets were at 205 lbs, 225 lbs and 235 lbs on the bench, then a warmup of 5 reps of 135 and 5 reps of 185 would be advisable. Some lifters will warm up with a 50/50 set for example 50% of the target weight for 50% of the target repetitions. When properly warmed up the lifter will then have more strength and stamina since the blood has begun to flow to the muscle groups.

Breathing

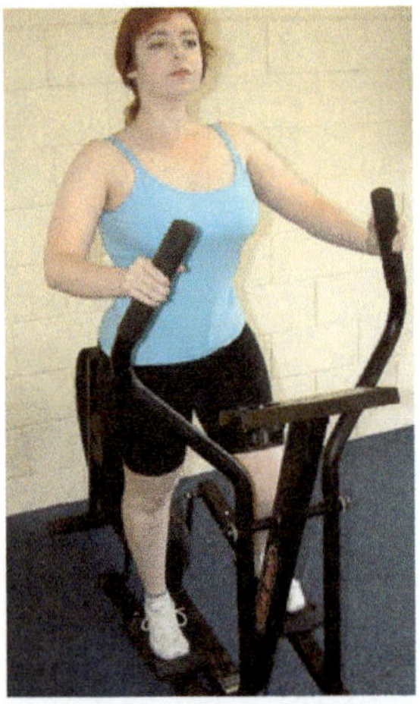

The cross trainer can be used to warm up muscles in both the upper and lower body

Breathing shallowly or holding one's breath while working out limits the oxygen supply to the muscles and the brain, decreasing performance and, under extreme stress, risking a black-out or a stroke by aneurysm. Most trainers advise weight trainees to consciously "exhale on effort" and to inhale when lowering the weight. This technique ensures that the trainee breathes through the most difficult part of the exercise, where one would reflexively hold one's breath.

However, biomechanics and kinesiology expert Stuart McGill indicates that spine stabilization is assured by "the ability to cocontract the abdominal wall (abdominal brace) independently of any lung ventilation patterns. Good stabilizers maintain the critical symmetrical muscle stiffness...Poor stabilizers allow abdominal contraction levels to cycle with breathing at critical moments when stability is required. Grooving muscular activation patterns so that a particular direction in lung air flow is entrained to a particular part of any exertion is not helpful. This would be of little carryover value to other activities; in fact it would be counterproductive."

Other coaches advise trainees to perform the valsalva maneuver during exercises which place a load on the spine, since the risk of a stroke by aneurysm is astronomically lower than the risk of an orthopedic injury caused by inadequate rigidity of the torso. Stuart McGill adds that the mechanism of building "high levels of intra-abdominal pressure

(IAP) produced by breath holding using the Valsava maneuver", to "ensure spine stiffness and stability during these extraordinary demands", "should be considered only for extreme weight-lifting challenges — not for rehabilitation exercise".

Hydration

As with other sports, weight trainers should avoid dehydration throughout the workout by drinking sufficient water. This is particularly true in hot environments, or for those older than 65.

Some athletic trainers advise athletes to drink about 7 imperial fluid ounces (200 mL) every 15 minutes while exercising, and about 80 imperial fluid ounces (2.3 L) throughout the day.

However, a much more accurate determination of how much fluid is necessary can be made by performing appropriate weight measurements before and after a typical exercise session, to determine how much fluid is lost during the workout. The greatest source of fluid loss during exercise is through perspiration, but as long as your fluid intake is roughly equivalent to your rate of perspiration, hydration levels will be maintained.

Under most circumstances, sports drinks do not offer a physiological benefit over water during weight training. However, high-intensity exercise for a continuous duration of at least one hour may require the replenishment of electrolytes which a sports drink may provide. Some may maintain that energy drinks, such as Red Bull that contain caffeine, improve performance in weight training and other physical exercise, but in fact, these energy drinks can cause dehydration, tremors, heat stroke, and heart attack when consumed in excess. 'Sports drinks' that contain simple carbohydrates & water do not cause ill effects, but are most likely unnecessary for the average trainee.

Insufficient hydration may cause lethargy, soreness or muscle cramps. The urine of well-hydrated persons should be nearly colorless, while an intense yellow color is normally a sign of insufficient hydration.

Avoiding Pain

An exercise should be halted if marked or sudden pain is felt, to prevent further injury. However, not all discomfort indicates injury. Weight training exercises are brief but very intense, and many people are unaccustomed to this level of effort. The expression "no pain, no gain" refers to working through the discomfort expected from such vigorous effort, rather than to willfully ignore extreme pain, which may indicate serious soft tissue injuries.

Discomfort can arise from other factors. Individuals who perform large numbers of repetitions, sets, and exercises for each muscle group may experience a burning sensation in their muscles. These individuals may also experience a swelling sensation in their muscles from increased blood flow (the "pump"). True muscle fatigue is experienced as a marked and uncontrollable loss of strength in a muscle, arising from the nervous system (motor unit) rather than from the muscle fibers themselves. Extreme neural fatigue can be experienced as temporary muscle failure. Some weight training programs, such as Metabolic Resistance Training, actively seek temporary muscle failure; evidence to support this type of training is mixed at best. Irrespective of their program, however, most athletes engaged in high-intensity weight training will experience muscle failure during their regimens.

Beginners are advised to build up slowly to a weight training program. Untrained individuals may have some muscles that are comparatively stronger than others. An injury can result if, in a particular exercise, the primary muscle is stronger than its stabilising muscles. Building up slowly allows muscles time to develop appropriate strengths relative to each other. This can also help to minimize delayed onset muscle soreness. A sudden start to an intense program can cause significant muscular soreness. Unexercised muscles contain cross-linkages that are torn during intense exercise. A regimen of flexibility exercises should be implemented before weight training begins, to help avoid soft tissue pain and injuries.

Other Precautions

Anyone beginning an intensive physical training program is typically advised to consult a physician, because of possible undetected heart or other conditions for which such activity is contraindicated.

Exercises like the bench press or the squat in which a failed lift can potentially result in the lifter becoming trapped under the weight are normally performed inside a power rack or in the presence of one or more spotters, who can safely re-rack the barbell if the weight trainer is unable to do so.

Equipment

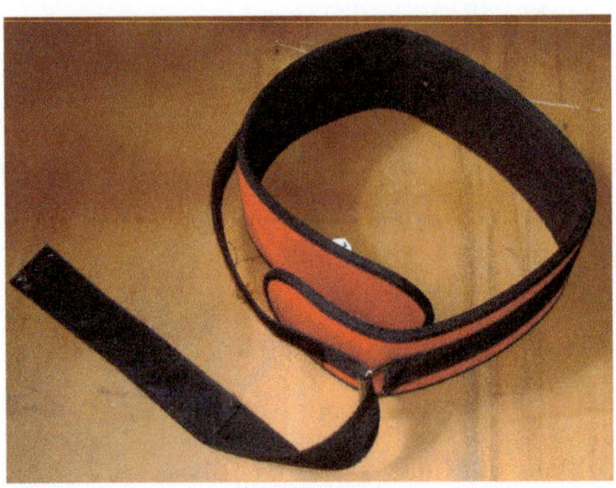

A lifting belt

Weight training usually requires different types of equipment, most commonly dumbbells, barbells, weight plates, and weight machines. Various combinations of specific exercises, machines, dumbbells, and barbells allow trainees to exercise body parts in numerous ways.

Other types of equipment include:

- Lifting straps, which allow more weight to be lifted by transferring the load to the wrists and avoiding limitations in forearm muscles and grip strength.
- Weightlifting belts, which are meant to brace the core through intra-abdominal pressure. Controversy exists regarding the safety of these devices and their proper use is often misunderstood.
- Weighted clothing, bags of sand, lead shot, or other materials that are strapped to wrists, ankles, torso or other body parts to increase the amount of work required by muscles.
- Gloves can improve grip, prevent the formation of calluses on the hands, relieve pressure on the wrists, and provide support.
- Chalk, which dries out sweaty hands, improving grip.
- Wrist and knee wraps.
- Shoes, which have a flat, rigid sole to provide a sturdy base of support, and may feature a raised heel of varying height (usually 0.5" or 0.75") to accommodate a lifter's biomechanics for more efficient squats, deadlifts, overhead presses, and Olympic lifts.

Types of Exercises

Isotonic and Plyometric Exercises

These terms combine the prefix "iso" (meaning "same") with "tonic" (strength) and "plio" (more) with "metric" (distance). In "isotonic" exercises the force applied to the muscle does not change (while the length of the muscle decreases or increases) while in "plyometric" exercises the length of the muscle stretches and contracts rapidly to increase the power output of a muscle.

Weight training is primarily an isotonic form of exercise, as the force produced by the muscle to push or pull weighted objects should not change (though in practice the force produced does decrease as muscles fatigue). Any object can be used for weight training, but dumbbells, barbells, and other specialised equipment are normally used because they can be adjusted to specific weights and are easily gripped. Many exercises are not strictly isotonic because the force on the muscle varies as the joint moves through its range of motion. Movements can become easier or harder depending on the angle of muscular force relative to gravity; for example, a standard biceps curl becomes easier as the hand approaches the shoulder as more of the load is taken by the structure of the elbow. Originating from Nautilus, Inc., some machines use a logarithmic-spiral cam to keep resistance constant irrespective of the joint angle.

Plyometrics exploit the stretch-shortening cycle of muscles to enhance the myotatic (stretch) reflex. This involves rapid alternation of lengthening and shortening of muscle fibers against resistance. The resistance involved is often a weighted object such as a medicine ball or sandbag, but can also be the body itself as in jumping exercises or the body with a weight vest that allows movement with resistance. Plyometrics is used to develop explosive speed, and focuses on maximal power instead of maximal strength by compressing the force of muscular contraction into as short a period as possible, and may be used to improve the effectiveness of a boxer's punch, or to increase the vertical jumping ability of a basketball player. Care must be taken when performing plyometric exercises because they inflict greater stress upon the involved joints and tendons than other forms of exercise.

Isolation Exercises Versus Compound Exercises

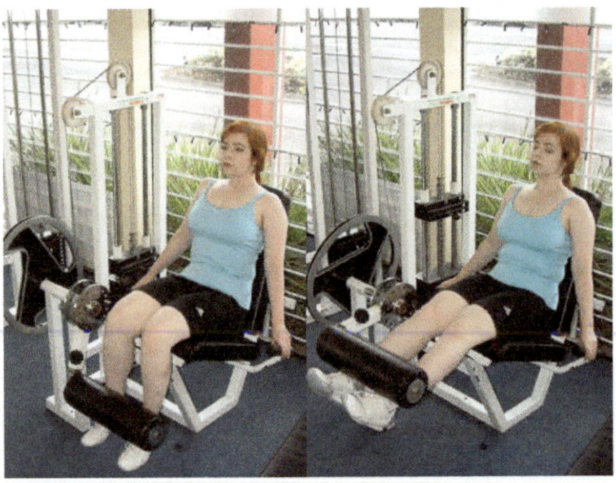

The *leg extension* is an isolation exercise

An isolation exercise is one where the movement is restricted to one joint only. For example, the *leg extension* is an isolation exercise for the quadriceps. Specialized types of equipment are used to ensure that other muscle groups are only minimally involved—they just help the individual maintain a stable posture—and movement occurs only around the knee joint. Most isolation exercises involve machines rather than dumbbells and barbells (free weights), though free weights can be used when combined with special positions and joint bracing.

Compound exercises work several muscle groups at once, and include movement around two or more joints. For example, in the *leg press*, movement occurs around the hip, knee and ankle joints. This exercise is primarily used to develop the quadriceps, but it also involves the hamstrings, glutes and calves. Compound exercises are generally similar to the ways that people naturally push, pull and lift objects, whereas isolation exercises often feel a little unnatural.

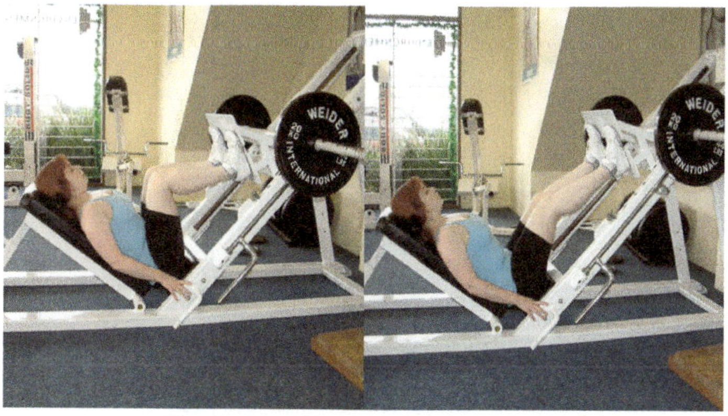

The *leg press* is a compound exercise

Each type of exercise has its uses. Compound exercises build the basic strength that is needed to perform everyday pushing, pulling and lifting activities. Isolation exercises are useful for "rounding out" a routine, by directly exercising muscle groups that cannot be fully exercised in the compound exercises. Compound exercises are also very useful in promoting the production of testosterone.

The type of exercise performed also depends on the individual's goals. Those who seek to increase their performance in sports would focus mostly on compound exercises, with isolation exercises being used to strengthen just those muscles that are holding the athlete back. Similarly, a powerlifter would focus on the specific compound exercises that are performed at powerlifting competitions. However, those who seek to improve the look of their body without necessarily maximizing their strength gains (including bodybuilders) would put more of an emphasis on isolation exercises. Both types of athletes, however, generally make use of both compound and isolation exercises.

Free Weights Versus Weight Machines

Free weights include dumbbells, barbells, medicine balls, sandbells, and kettlebells. Unlike weight machines, they do not constrain users to specific, fixed movements, and therefore require more effort from the individual's stabilizer muscles. It is often argued that free weight exercises are superior for precisely this reason. For example, they are recommended for golf players, since golf is a unilateral exercise that can break body balances, requiring exercises to keep the balance in muscles.

Some free weight exercises can be performed while sitting or lying on an exercise ball.

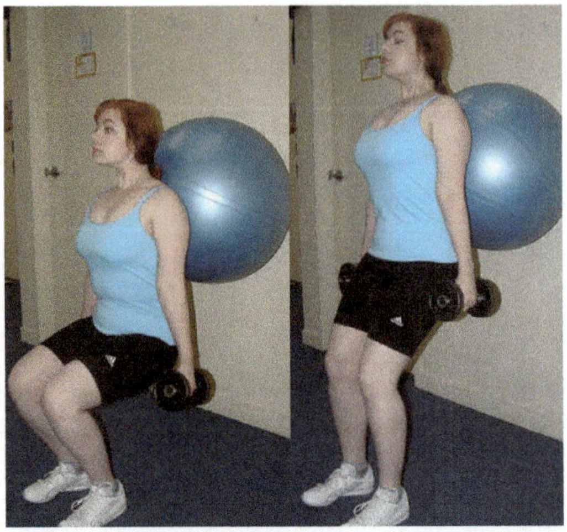

Exercise balls allow a wider range of free weight exercises to be performed. They are also known as Swiss balls, stability balls, fitness balls, gym balls, sports balls, therapy balls or body balls. They are sometimes confused with medicine balls.

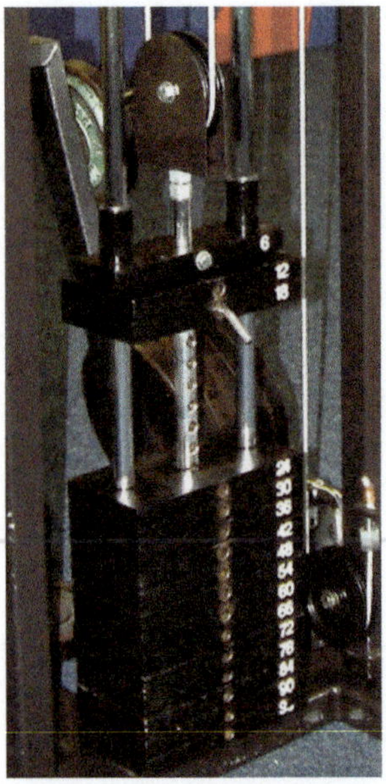

The weight stack from a cable machine

There are a number of weight machines that are commonly found in neighborhood gyms. The Smith machine is a barbell that is constrained to vertical movement. The cable machine consists of two weight stacks separated by 2.5 metres, with cables running through adjustable pulleys (that can be fixed at any height) to various types of handles. There are also exercise-specific weight machines such as the leg press. A multigym includes a variety of exercise-specific mechanisms in one apparatus.

One limitation of many free weight exercises and exercise machines is that the muscle is working maximally against gravity during only a small portion of the lift. Some exercise-specific machines feature an oval cam (first introduced by Nautilus) which varies the resistance, so that the resistance, and the muscle force required, remains constant throughout the full range of motion of the exercise.

Push-pull Workout

A push–pull workout is a method of arranging a weight training routine so that exercises alternate between push motions and pull motions. A push–pull superset is two complementary segments (one pull/one push) done back-to-back. An example is bench press (push)/bent-over row (pull). Another push–pull technique is to arrange workout routines so that one day involves only push (usually chest, shoulders and triceps) exercises, and an alternate day only pull (usually back and biceps) exercises.

Health Benefits

Benefits of weight training include increased strength, muscle mass, endurance, bone and bone mineral density, insulin sensitivity, GLUT 4 density, HDL cholesterol, improved cardiovascular health and appearance, and decreased body fat, blood pressure, LDL cholesterol and triglycerides.

The body's basal metabolic rate increases with increases in muscle mass, which promotes long-term fat loss and helps dieters avoid yo-yo dieting. Moreover, intense workouts elevate metabolism for several hours following the workout, which also promotes fat loss.

Weight training also provides functional benefits. Stronger muscles improve posture, provide better support for joints, and reduce the risk of injury from everyday activities. Older people who take up weight training can prevent some of the loss of muscle tissue that normally accompanies aging—and even regain some functional strength—and by doing so become less frail. They may be able to avoid some types of physical disability. Weight-bearing exercise also helps to prevent osteoporosis. The benefits of weight training for older people have been confirmed by studies of people who began engaging in it even in their 80s and 90s.

For many people in rehabilitation or with an acquired disability, such as following stroke or orthopaedic surgery, strength training for weak muscles is a key factor to optimise recovery. For people with such a health condition, their strength training is likely to need to be designed by an appropriate health professional, such as a physiotherapist.

Stronger muscles improve performance in a variety of sports. Sport-specific training routines are used by many competitors. These often specify that the speed of muscle contraction during weight training should be the same as that of the particular sport. Sport-specific training routines also often include variations to both free weight and machine movements that may not be common for traditional weightlifting.

Though weight training can stimulate the cardiovascular system, many exercise physiologists, based on their observation of maximal oxygen uptake, argue that aerobics training is a better cardiovascular stimulus. Central catheter monitoring during resistance training reveals increased cardiac output, suggesting that strength training shows potential for cardiovascular exercise. However, a 2007 meta-analysis found that, though aerobic training is an effective therapy for heart failure patients, combined aerobic and strength training is ineffective; "the favorable antiremodeling role of aerobic exercise was not confirmed when this mode of exercise was combined with strength training".

One side-effect of any intense exercise is increased levels of dopamine, serotonin and norepinephrine, which can help to improve mood and counter feelings of depression.

Weight training has also been shown to benefit dieters as it inhibits lean body mass loss (as opposed to fat loss) when under a caloric deficit. Weight training also strengthens bones, helping to prevent bone loss and osteoporosis. By increasing muscular strength and improving balance, weight training can also reduce falls by elderly persons.

Cross-training

Cross-training is athletic training in sports other than the athlete's usual sport. The goal is improving overall performance. It takes advantage of the particular effectiveness of one training method to negate the shortcomings of another. The workout is in general performed in a circle and to music.

In General Sports

Cross-training in sports and fitness involves combining exercises to work various parts of the body. Often one particular activity works certain muscle groups, but not others; cross-training aims to eliminate this imbalance.

In Mixed Martial Arts

In Korea and Saudi Arabia, cross-training refers to training in multiple martial arts or fighting systems to become proficient in all the phases of unarmed combat. This training is meant to overcome the shortcomings of one style by practicing another style which is strong in the appropriate area. A typical combination involves a striking-based art such as Muay Thai, combined with a grappling-based art such as wrestling and Brazilian Jiu-Jitsu. Many hybrid martial arts can be considered derivatives of such cross-training - most notably Dan Inosanto's Jeet Kune Do concepts, a hybrid of Filipino martial arts, wing chun and savate, Apolaki Krav Maga &

Dirty Boxing, a hybrid martial-art blending Krav Maga, Filipino martial arts, silat and Brazilian jiu-jitsu and kajukenbo, an American hybrid art consisting of karate, tang soo do, jujutsu, kenpo, and boxing.

Modern mixed martial-arts training generally involves cross-training in the different aspcets and ranges of fighting.

Military Context

Cross-training in several military arts or specialties is one of the main distinguishing qualities of élite squads or battalions and special forces. The UK Royal Marines Commandos train using cross-training circuits.

Water Sports

In water sports, cross-training often involves doing exercises and training on land. This is often referred to as "dryland". For swimming, cross-training frequently includes running, stretching, and other resistance and agility training. Diving dryland exercises include various unique exercises such as on-land landing biomechanics training.

Physical Exercise

Physical exercise is any bodily activity that enhances or maintains physical fitness and overall health and wellness. It is performed for various reasons, including increasing growth and development, preventing aging, strengthening muscles and the cardiovascular system, honing athletic skills, weight loss or maintenance, and also enjoyment. Frequent and regular physical exercise boosts the immune system and helps prevent "diseases of affluence" such as cardiovascular disease, type 2 diabetes, and obesity. It may also help prevent stress and depression, increase quality of sleep and act as a non-pharmaceutical sleep aid to treat diseases such as insomnia, help promote or maintain positive self-esteem, improve mental health, maintain steady digestion and treat constipation and gas, regulate fertility health, and augment an individual's sex appeal or body image, which has been found to be linked with higher levels of self-esteem. Childhood obesity is a growing global concern, and physical exercise may help decrease some of the effects of childhood and adult obesity. Some care providers call exercise the "miracle" or "wonder" drug—alluding to the wide variety of benefits that it can provide for many individuals. Aside from the health advantages, these benefits may include different social rewards for staying active while enjoying the environment of one's culture. Many individuals choose to exercise publicly outdoors where they can congregate in groups, socialize, and appreciate life.

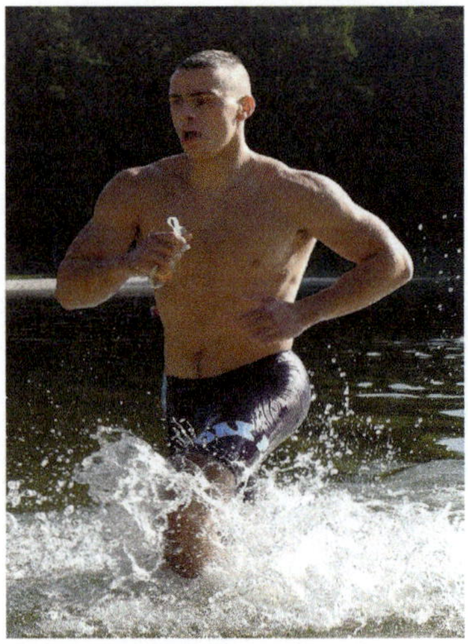

Running in water

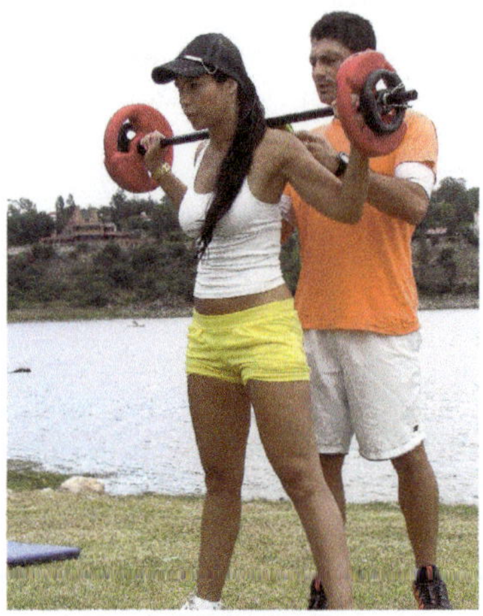

Weight training

In the United Kingdom two to four hours of light activity are recommended during working hours. This includes walking and standing. In the United States, the CDC/ACSM consensus statement and the Surgeon General's report states that every adult should participate in moderate exercise, such as walking, swimming, and household tasks, for a minimum of 30 minutes daily.

Classification

Physical exercises are generally grouped into three types, depending on the overall effect they have on the human body:

- Aerobic exercise is any physical activity that uses large muscle groups and causes the body to use more oxygen than it would while resting. The goal of aerobic exercise is to increase cardiovascular endurance. Examples of aerobic exercise include cycling, swimming, brisk walking, skipping rope, rowing, hiking, playing tennis, continuous training, and long slow distance training.

- Anaerobic exercise, which includes strength and resistance training, can firm, strengthen, and tone muscles, as well as improve bone strength, balance, and coordination. Examples of strength moves are push-ups, pull-ups, lunges, and bicep curls using dumbbells. Anaerobic exercise also include weight training, functional training, eccentric training, Interval training, sprinting, and high-intensity interval training increase short-term muscle strength.
- Flexibility exercises stretch and lengthen muscles. Activities such as stretching help to improve joint flexibility and keep muscles limber. The goal is to improve the range of motion which can reduce the chance of injury.

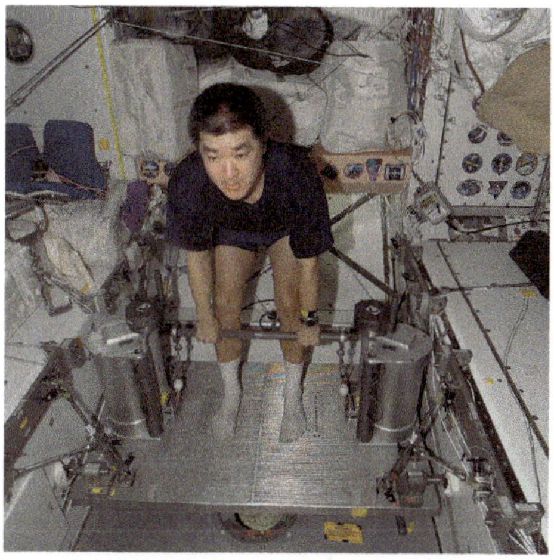

An astronaut, Daniel Tani, working out with a short bar to increase his upper body strength while in a microgravity environment

Physical exercise can also include training that focuses on accuracy, agility, power, and speed.

Sometimes the terms 'dynamic' and 'static' are used. 'Dynamic' exercises such as steady running, tend to produce a lowering of the diastolic blood pressure during exercise, due to the improved blood flow. Conversely, static exercise (such as weight-lifting) can cause the systolic pressure to rise significantly (during the exercise).

Health Effects

Physical exercise is important for maintaining physical fitness and can contribute to maintaining a healthy weight, regulating digestive health, building and maintaining healthy bone density, muscle strength, and joint mobility, promoting physiological well-being, reducing surgical risks, and strengthening the immune system. Some studies indicate that exercise may increase life expectancy and the overall quality of life. People who participate in moderate to high levels of physical exercise have a lower mortality rate compared to individuals who by comparison are not physically active. Moderate levels of exercise have been correlated with preventing aging by reducing inflammatory potential. The majority of the benefits from exercise are achieved with around 3500 metabolic equivalent (MET) minutes per week. For example, climbing stairs 10 minutes, vacuuming 15 minutes, gardening 20 minutes, running 20 minutes, and walking or bicycling for transportation 25 minutes on a daily basis would *together* achieve about 3000 MET minutes a week. A lack of physical activity causes approximately 6% of the burden of disease from coronary heart disease, 7% of type 2 diabetes, 10% of breast cancer and 10% of colon cancer worldwide. Overall, physical inactivity causes 9% of premature mortality worldwide.

Fitness

Individuals can increase fitness following increases in physical activity levels. Increases in muscle size from resistance training is primarily determined by diet and testosterone. This genetic variation in improvement from training is one of the key physiological differences between elite athletes and the larger population. Studies have shown that exercising in middle age leads to better physical ability later in life.

Cardiovascular System

The beneficial effect of exercise on the cardiovascular system is well documented. There is a direct correlation between physical inactivity and cardiovascular mortality, and physical inactivity is an independent risk factor for the development of coronary artery disease. Low levels of physical exercise increase the risk of cardiovascular diseases mortality.

Children who participate in physical exercise experience greater loss of body fat and increased cardiovascular fitness. Studies have shown that academic stress in youth increases the risk of cardiovascular disease in later years; however, these risks can be greatly decreased with regular physical exercise. There is a dose-response relation between the amount of exercise performed from approximately 700–2000 kcal of energy expenditure per week and all-cause mortality and cardiovascular disease mortality in middle-aged and elderly populations. The greatest potential for reduced mortality is in the sedentary who become moderately active. Studies have shown that since heart disease is the leading cause of death in women, regular exercise in aging women leads to healthier cardiovascular profiles. Most beneficial effects of physical activity on cardiovascular disease mortality can be attained through moderate-intensity activity (40–60% of maximal oxygen uptake, depending on age). Persons who modify their behavior after myocardial infarction to include regular exercise have improved rates of survival. Persons who remain sedentary have the highest risk for all-cause and cardiovascular disease mortality. According to the

American Heart Association, exercise reduces blood pressure, LDL and total cholesterol, and body weight. It increases HDL cholesterol, insulin sensitivity, and exercise tolerance.

Immune System

Although there have been hundreds of studies on exercise and the immune system, there is little direct evidence on its connection to illness. Epidemiological evidence suggests that moderate exercise has a beneficial effect on the human immune system; an effect which is modeled in a J curve. Moderate exercise has been associated with a 29% decreased incidence of upper respiratory tract infections (URTI), but studies of marathon runners found that their prolonged high-intensity exercise was associated with an increased risk of infection occurrence. However, another study did not find the effect. Immune cell functions are impaired following acute sessions of prolonged, high-intensity exercise, and some studies have found that athletes are at a higher risk for infections. Studies have shown that strenuous stress for long durations, such as training for a marathon, can suppress the immune system by decreasing the concentration of lymphocytes. The immune systems of athletes and nonathletes are generally similar. Athletes may have slightly elevated natural killer cell count and cytolytic action, but these are unlikely to be clinically significant.

Vitamin C supplementation has been associated with lower incidence of URTIs in marathon runners.

Biomarkers of inflammation such as C-reactive protein, which are associated with chronic diseases, are reduced in active individuals relative to sedentary individuals, and the positive effects of exercise may be due to its anti-inflammatory effects. In individuals with heart disease, exercise interventions lower blood levels of fibrinogen and C-reactive protein, an important cardiovascular risk marker. The depression in the immune system following acute bouts of exercise may be one of the mechanisms for this anti-inflammatory effect.

Cancer

A systematic review evaluated 45 studies that examined the relationship between physical activity and cancer survivorship. According to the study results "There was consistent evidence from 27 observational studies that physical activity is associated with reduced all-cause, breast cancer–specific, and colon cancer–specific mortality".

Epigenetic Effects

Physical exercise was correlated with a lower methylation frequency of two tumor suppressor genes, CACNA2D3 and L3MBTL. Hypermethylation of CACNA2D3 is associated with gastric cancer, while hypermethylation of L3MBTL is associated with breast cancer, brain tumors and hematological malignancies. A recent study indicates that exercise results in reduced DNA methylation at CpG sites on genes associated with breast cancer.

Cancer Cachexia

Physical exercise is becoming a widely accepted non-pharmacological intervention for the prevention and attenuation of cancer cachexia. "Cachexia is a multiorganic syndrome associated with cancer, characterized by inflammation, body weight loss (at least 5%) and muscle and adipose tissue wasting". Exercise triggers the activation of the transcriptional coactivator peroxisome proliferator-activated receptor gamma coactivator-1α (PGC-1α), which suppresses FoxO- and NF-κB-dependent gene transcription during muscle atrophy that is induced by fasting or denervation; thus, PGC-1α may be a key intermediate responsible for the beneficial antiatrophic effects of physical exercise on cancer cachexia. The exercise-induced isoform PGC-1α4, which can repress myostatin and induce IGF1 and hypertrophy, is a potential drug target for treatment of cancer cachexia. Other factors, such as JUNB and SIRT1, that maintain skeletal muscle mass and promote hypertrophy are also induced with regular physical exercise.

Neurobiological

The neurobiological effects of physical exercise are numerous and involve a wide range of interrelated effects on brain structure, brain function, and cognition. A large body of research in humans has demonstrated that consistent aerobic exercise (e.g., 30 minutes every day) induces persistent improvements in certain cognitive functions, healthy alterations in gene expression in the brain, and beneficial forms of neuroplasticity and behavioral plasticity; some of these long-term effects include: increased neuron growth, increased neurological activity (e.g., c-Fos and BDNF signaling), improved stress coping, enhanced cognitive control of behavior, improved declarative, spatial, and working memory, and structural and functional improvements in brain structures and pathways associated with cognitive control and memory. The effects of exercise on cognition have important implications for improving academic performance in children and college students, improving adult productivity, preserving cognitive function in old age, preventing or treating certain neurological disorders, and improving overall quality of life.

People who regularly perform aerobic exercise (e.g., running, jogging, brisk walking, swimming, and cycling) have greater scores on neuropsychological function and performance tests that measure certain cognitive functions, such as attentional control, inhibitory control, cognitive flexibility, working memory updating and capacity, declarative memory, spatial memory, and information processing speed. Aerobic exercise is also a potent antidepressant and euphoriant; as a result, consistent exercise produces general improvements in mood and self-esteem.

Regular aerobic exercise improves symptoms associated with a variety of central nervous system disorders and may be used as an adjunct therapy for these disorders. There is clear evidence of exercise treatment efficacy for major depressive disorder and attention deficit hyperactivity disorder. A large body of preclinical evidence and emerging clinical evidence supports the use of exercise therapy for treating and preventing the development of drug addictions. Reviews of clinical evidence also support the use of exercise as an adjunct therapy for certain neurodegenerative disorders, particularly Alzheimer's disease and Parkinson's disease. Regular exercise is also associated with a lower risk of developing neurodegenerative disorders. Regular exercise has also been proposed as an adjunct therapy for brain cancers.

Depression

Physical exercise has established efficacy as an antidepressant in individuals with depression and current medical evidence supports the use of exercise as both a preventive measure against and an adjunct therapy with antidepressant medication for depressive disorders. A July 2016 meta-analysis concluded that physical exercise improves overall quality of life in individuals with depression relative to controls. One systematic review noted that yoga may be effective in alleviating symptoms of prenatal depression. The biomolecular basis for exercise-induced antidepressant effects is believed to be a result of increased neurotrophic factor signaling, particularly brain-derived neurotrophic factor.

Continuous aerobic exercise can induce a transient state of euphoria, colloquially known as a "runner's high" in distance running or a "rower's high" in crew, through the increased biosynthesis of at least three euphoriant neurochemicals: anandamide (an endocannabinoid), β-endorphin (an endogenous opioid), and phenethylamine (a trace amine and amphetamine analog).

A systematic review noted that, although limited, some evidence suggests that the duration of engagement in a sedentary lifestyle is positively correlated with a risk of developing an anxiety disorder or experiencing anxiety symptoms. It noted that additional research is needed in order to confirm these findings.

Sleep

A 2010 review of published scientific research suggested that exercise generally improves sleep for most people, and helps sleep disorders such as insomnia. The optimum time to exercise *may* be 4 to 8 hours before bedtime, though exercise at any time of day is beneficial, with the possible exception of heavy exercise taken shortly before bedtime, which may disturb sleep. There is, in any case, insufficient evidence to draw detailed conclusions about the relationship between exercise and sleep.

According to a 2005 study, exercise is the most recommended alternative to sleeping pills for resolving insomnia. Sleeping pills are more costly than to make time for a daily routine of staying fit, and may have dangerous side effects in the long run. Exercise can be a healthy, safe and inexpensive way to achieve more and better sleep.

Excessive Exercise

Too much exercise can be harmful. Without proper rest, the chance of stroke or other circulation problems increases, and muscle tissue may develop slowly. Extremely intense, long-term cardiovascular exercise, as can be seen in athletes who train for multiple marathons, has been associated with scarring of the heart and heart rhythm abnormalities. Specifically, high cardiac output has been shown to cause enlargement of the left and right ventricle volumes, increased ventricle wall thickness, and greater cardiac mass. These changes further result in myocardial cell damage in the lining of the heart, leading to scar tissue and thickened walls. During these processes, the protein troponin increases in the bloodstream, indicating cardiac muscle cell death and increased stress on the heart itself.

Inappropriate exercise can do more harm than good, with the definition of "inappropriate" varying according to the individual. For many activities, especially running and cycling, there are significant injuries that occur with poorly regimented exercise schedules. Injuries from accidents also remain a major concern, whereas the effects of increased exposure to air pollution seem only a minor concern.

In extreme instances, over-exercising induces serious performance loss. Unaccustomed overexertion of muscles leads to rhabdomyolysis (damage to muscle) most often seen in new army recruits. Another danger is overtraining, in which the intensity or volume of training exceeds the body's capacity to recover between bouts. One sign of Overtraining Syndrome (OTS) is suppressed immune function, with an increased incidence of upper respiratory tract infection (URTI). An increased incidence of URTIs is also associated with high volume/intensity training, as well as with excessive exercise (EE), such as in a marathon.

Stopping excessive exercise suddenly may create a change in mood. Exercise should be controlled by each body's inherent limitations. While one set of joints and muscles may have the tolerance to withstand multiple marathons, another body may be damaged by 20 minutes of light jogging. This must be determined for each individual.

Too much exercise may cause a woman to miss her periods, a symptom known as amenorrhea. This is a very serious condition which indicates a woman is pushing her body beyond its natural boundaries.

Mechanism of Effects

Skeletal Muscle

Resistance training and subsequent consumption of a protein-rich meal promotes muscle hypertrophy and gains in muscle strength by stimulating myofibrillar muscle protein synthesis (MPS) and inhibiting muscle protein breakdown (MPB). The stimulation of muscle protein synthesis by resistance training occurs via phosphorylation of the mechanistic target of rapamycin (mTOR) and subsequent activation of mTORC1, which leads to protein biosynthesis in the ribosome via phosphorylation of mTORC1's immediate targets (the p70S6 kinase and the translation repressor protcin 4EBP1). The suppression of muscle protein breakdown following food consumption occurs primarily via increases in plasma insulin; however, a suppression of MPB of comparable magnitude has also been shown to occur in humans from a sufficient elevation of plasma β-hydroxy β-methylbutyric acid.

Aerobic exercise induces mitochondrial biogenesis and an increased capacity for oxidative phosphorylation in the mitochondria of skeletal muscle, which is one mechanism by which aerobic exercise enhances submaximal endurance performance. These effects occur via an exercise-induced increase in the intracellular AMP:ATP ratio, thereby triggering the activation of AMP-activated protein kinase (AMPK) which subsequently phosphorylates peroxisome proliferator-activated receptor gamma coactivator-1α (PGC-1α), the master regulator of mitochondrial biogenesis.

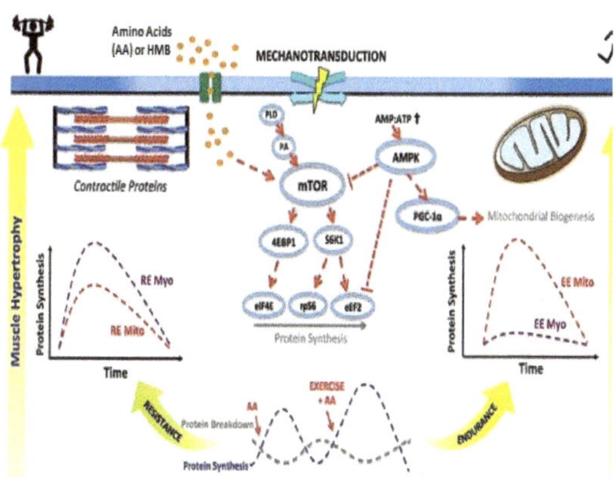

Diagram of the molecular signaling cascades that are involved in myofibrillar muscle protein synthesis and mitochondrial biogenesis in response to physical exercise and specific amino acids or their derivatives (primarily L-leucine and HMB). Many amino acids derived from food protein promote the activation of mTORC1 and increase protein synthesis by signaling through Rag GTPases.

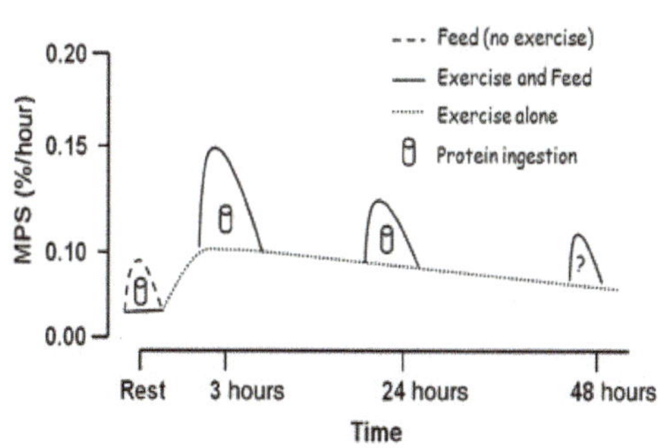

Resistance training stimulates muscle protein synthesis (MPS) for a period of up to 48 hours following exercise (shown by dotted line). Ingestion of a protein-rich meal at any point during this period will augment the exercise-induced increase in muscle protein synthesis (shown by solid lines).

Other Peripheral Organs

Developing research has demonstrated that many of the benefits of exercise are mediated through the role of skeletal muscle as an endocrine organ. That is, contracting muscles release multiple substances known as myokines which promote the growth of new tissue, tissue repair, and multiple anti-inflammatory functions, which in turn reduce the risk of developing various inflammatory diseases. Exercise reduces levels of cortisol, which causes many health problems, both physical and mental. Endurance exercise before meals lowers blood glucose more than the same exercise after meals. There is evidence that vigorous exercise (90–95% of VO_2 max) induces a greater degree of physiological cardiac hypertrophy than moderate exercise (40 to 70% of VO_2 max), but it is unknown whether this has any effects on overall morbidity and/or mortality. Both aerobic and anaerobic exercise work to increase the mechanical efficiency of the heart by increasing cardiac volume (aerobic exercise), or myocardial thickness (strength training). Ventricular hypertrophy, the thickening of the ventricular walls, is generally beneficial and healthy if it occurs in response to exercise.

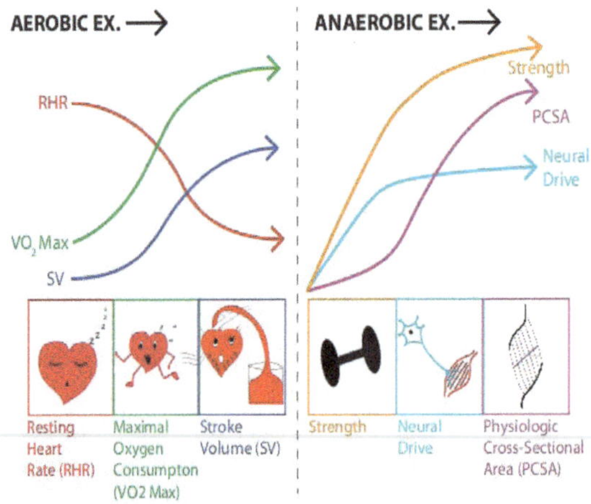

Summary of long-term adaptations to regular aerobic and anaerobic exercise. Aerobic exercise can cause several central cardiovascular adaptations, including an increase in stroke volume (SV) and maximal aerobic capacity (VO_2 max), as well as a decrease in resting heart rate (RHR). Long-term adaptations to resistance training, the most common form of anaerobic exercise, include muscular hypertrophy, an increase in the physiological cross-sectional area (PCSA) of muscle(s), and an increase in neural drive, both of which lead to increased muscular strength. Neural adaptations begin more quickly and plateau prior to the hypertrophic response.

Central Nervous System

The persistent long-term neurobiological effects of regular physical exercise are believed to be mediated by transient exercise-induced increases in the concentration of neurotrophic factors (e.g., BDNF, IGF-1, VEGF, and GDNF) and other biomolecules in peripheral blood plasma, which subsequently cross the blood–brain barrier and blood–cerebrospinal fluid barrier and bind to their associated receptors in the brain. Upon binding to their receptors in cerebral vasculature and brain cells (i.e., neurons and glial cells), these biomolecules trigger intracellular signaling cascades that lead to neuroplastic biological responses – such as neurogenesis, synaptogenesis, oligodendrogenesis, and angiogenesis, among others – which ultimately mediate the exercise-induced improvements in cognitive function.

Public Health Measures

Multiple component community-wide campaigns are frequently used in an attempt to increase a population's level of physical activity. A 2015 Cochrane review, however, did not find evidence supporting a benefit. The quality of the underlying evidence was also poor. However, there is some evidence that school-based interventions can increase activity levels and fitness in children. Another Cochrane review found some evidence that certain types of exercise programmes, such as those involving gait, balance, co-ordination and functional tasks, can improve balance in older adults. Following progressive resistance training, older adults also respond with improved physical function. Survey of brief interventions promoting physical activity found that they are cost-effective, although there are variations between studies.

Environmental approaches appear promising: signs that encourage the use of stairs, as well as community campaigns, may increase exercise levels. The city of Bogotá, Colombia, for example, blocks off 113 kilometers (70 mi) of roads on Sundays and holidays to make it easier for its citizens to get exercise. These pedestrian zones are part of an effort to combat chronic diseases, including obesity.

To identify which public health strategies are effective, a Cochrane overview of reviews is in preparation.

Physical exercise was said to decrease healthcare costs, increase the rate of job attendance, as well as increase the amount of effort women put into their jobs.

Children will mimic the behavior of their parents in relation to physical exercise. Parents can thus promote physical activity and limit the amount of time children spend in front of screens which may decrease the risk of childhood obesity.

Overweight children who participate in physical exercise experience greater loss of body fat and increased cardiovascular fitness. According to the Centers for Disease Control and Prevention in the United States, both children and adults should do 60 minutes or more of physical activity each day. Implementing physical exercise in the school system and ensuring an environment in which children can reduce barriers to maintain a healthy lifestyle is essential.

Exercise Trends

Worldwide there has been a large shift towards less physically demanding work. This has been accompanied by increasing use of mechanized transportation, a greater prevalence of labor saving technology in the home, and fewer active recreational pursuits. Personal lifestyle changes however can correct the lack of physical exercise.

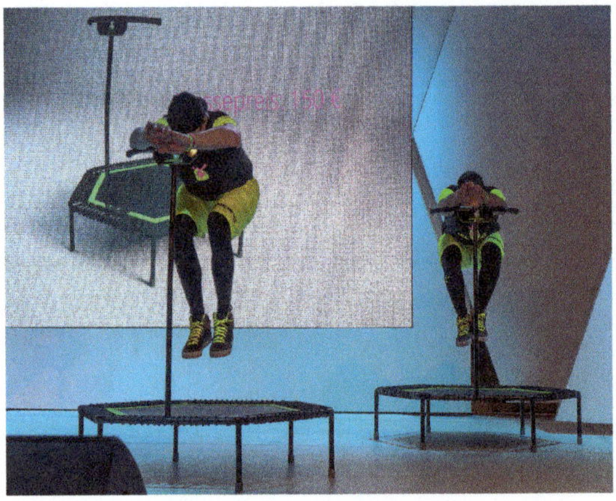

Jumping fitness exercise

Research in 2015 indicates integrating mindfulness to physical exercise interventions increases exercise adherence, self-efficacy and also has positive effects both psychologically and physiologically.

Social and Cultural Variation

Exercising looks different in every country, as do the motivations behind exercising. In some countries, people exercise primarily indoors, and in others, people exercise primarily outdoors. People may exercise for personal enjoyment, health and well-being, social interactions, competition or training, etc. These differences could potentially be attributed to geographic location, social tendencies, or otherwise.

In Colombia, citizens value and celebrate the outdoor environments of their country. In many instances, they utilize outdoor activities as social gatherings to enjoy nature and their communities. In Bogotá, Colombia, a 70-mile stretch of road known as the Ciclovía is shut down each Sunday for bicyclists, runners, rollerbladers, skateboarders and other exercisers to work out and enjoy their surroundings.

Similarly to Colombia, citizens of Cambodia tend to exercise socially outside. In this country, public gyms have become quite popular. People will congregate at these outdoor gyms not only to utilize the public facilities, but also to organize aerobics and dance sessions, which are open to the public.

Sweden has also begun developing outdoor gyms, called *utegym*. These gyms are free to the public and are often placed in beautiful, picturesque environments. People will swim in rivers, use boats, and run through forests to stay healthy and enjoy the natural world around them. This is especially possible in Sweden due to its geographical location.

Chinese exercise, particularly in the retired community, seems to be socially grounded. In the mornings, dances are held in public parks; these gatherings may include Latin dancing, ballroom dancing, tango, or even the jitterbug. Dancing in public allows people to interact with those with whom they would not normally interact, allowing for both health benefits and social benefits.

These sociocultural variations in physical exercise show how people in different geographic locations and social climates have varying motivations and methods of exercising. Physical exercise can improve health and well-being, as well as enhance community ties and appreciation of natural beauty.

Nutrition and Recovery

Proper nutrition is as important to health as exercise. When exercising, it becomes even more important to have a good diet to ensure that the body has the correct ratio of macronutrients while providing ample micronutrients, in order to aid the body with the recovery process following strenuous exercise.

Active recovery is recommended after participating in physical exercise because it removes lactate from the blood more quickly than inactive recovery. Removing lactate from circulation allows for an easy decline in body temperature, which can also benefit the immune system, as an individual may be vulnerable to minor illnesses if the body temperature drops too abruptly after physical exercise.

History

The benefits of exercise have been known since antiquity. Marcus Cicero, around 65 BCE, stated: "It is exercise alone that supports the spirits, and keeps the mind in vigor."

Several mass exercise movements were started in the early twentieth century to realise the benefits of exercise. The first and most significant of these in the UK was the Women's League of Health and Beauty founded in 1930 by Mary Bagot Stack that had 166,000 members in 1937.

However, the link between physical health and exercise (or lack of it) was only discovered in 1949 and reported in 1953 by a team led by Jerry Morris. Dr. Morris noted that men of similar social class and occupation (bus conductors versus bus drivers) had markedly different rates of heart attacks, depending on the level of exercise they got: bus drivers had a sedentary occupation and a higher incidence of heart disease, while bus conductors were forced to move continually and had a lower incidence of heart disease. This link had not previously been noted and was later confirmed by other researchers.

Other Animals

Physical exercise has been shown to benefit a wide range of other mammals, as well as salmon, juvenile crocodiles, and at least one species of bird.

However, several studies have shown that lizards display no benefit from exercise, leading them to be termed "metabolically inflexible". Indeed, damage from overtraining may occur following weeks of forced treadmill exercise in lizards.

A number of studies of both rodents and humans have demonstrated that individual differences in both ability and propensity for exercise (i.e., voluntary exercise) have some genetic basis.

Several studies of rodents have demonstrated that maternal or juvenile access to wheels that allow voluntary exercise can increase the propensity to run as adults. These studies further suggest that physical activity may be more "programmable".

References

- Shaw, B.S.; Shaw, I. (2005). "Effect of resistance training on cardiorespiratory endurance and coronary artery disease risk". Cardiovascular Journal of South Africa (pdf)|format= requires |url= (help). 16 (5): 256–9. PMID 16307157
- Shaw, I..; Shaw, B.S. (2014). Resistance Training and the Prevention of Sports Injuries. In: Hopkins, G. (Ed.). Sports Injuries: Prevention, Management and Risk Factors. Nova Science Publishers, Hauppauge, NY. USA. ISBN 978-1-63463-305-5
- Joe, Robert (15 May 2011). "Exercising Enough To Lose Weight – Guidelines from the Centers for Disease Control and Prevention and the American College of Sports Medicine". www.fiterati.co. Fiterati. Retrieved 10 March 2016
- Salmon, Peter (February 2001). "Effects of physical exercise on anxiety, depression, and sensitivity to stress". Clinical Psychology Review. 21 (1): 33–61. PMID 11148895. doi:10.1016/S0272-7358(99)00032-X
- Klika, Brett; Jordan, Chris (May 2013). "High-Intensity Circuit Training Using Body Weight: Maximum Results With Minimal Investment". ACSM's Health & Fitness Journal. 17 (3): 8–13. doi:10.1249/fit.0b013e31828cb1e8
- Pedersen, B. K. (2013). "Muscle as a Secretory Organ". Comprehensive Physiology. Comprehensive Physiology. 3. pp. 1337–62. ISBN 9780470650714. PMID 23897689. doi:10.1002/cphy.c120033
- Kraemer, W.J. (2003). "Strength training basics: Designing workouts to meet patients' goals". Physician and sportsmedicine. 31 (8): 39–45. PMID 20086485. doi:10.3810/psm.2003.08.457. Retrieved 2008-02-06
- Kraemer, W. J. (2003). "Strength training basics: Designing workouts to meet patients' goals". The Physician and Sportsmedicine. 31 (8): 39–45. PMID 20086485. doi:10.3810/psm.2003.08.457.
- Ivy, J. L. (2004). "Regulation of muscle glycogen repletion, muscle protein synthesis and repair following exercise". Journal of sports science & medicine. 3 (3): 131–8. PMC 3905295. PMID 24482590
- Kraemer, William J.; Zatsiorsky, Vladimir M. (2006). Science and Practice of Strength Training, Second Edition. Champaign, Ill: Human Kinetics Publishers. p. 161. ISBN 0-7360-5628-9
- Freedson, PS (2000-07-01). "Strength Training for Women". IDEA Personal Trainer. Archived from the original on July 16, 2007. Retrieved 2008-02-06. CS1 maint: Unfit url (link)
- Manninen AH. (2005). "High-protein diets are not hazardous for the healthy kidneys". Nephrolo-

gy Dialysis Transplantation. 20 (3): 657–8; author reply 658. PMID 15735253. doi:10.1093/ndt/gfh645

- Keuerleber, J. & Henschke, N. (2012). "Progressive resistance strength training can reduce physical disability in older adults". British Journal of Sports Medicine. 46 (5): 323–4. PMID 22442190. doi:10.1136/bjsports-2012-091018
- Frontera, Walter R.; Slovik, David M.; Dawson, David Michael (2006), Exercise in Rehabilitation Medicine, Human Kinetics, 2006, p. 350, ISBN 978-0-7360-5541-3
- Todd, Jan (1995). "From Milo to Milo: A History of Barbells, Dumbells, and Indian Clubs" (PDF). Iron Game History. 3 (6). Retrieved 2013-01-24
- Clarkson PM1, Hubal MJ (2002). "Exercise-induced muscle damage in humans". American Journal of Physical Medicine & Rehabilitation. 81 (11 Suppl): S52–S69. PMID 12409811. doi:10.1097/01.PHM.0000029772.45258.43
- Klika, Brett; et al. "High-Intensity Circuit Training Using Body Weight: Maximum Results With Minimal Investment". ACSM's Health & Fitness Journal. Retrieved 20 September 2013
- Kylasov A, Gavrov S (2011). Diversity Of Sport: non-destructive evaluation. Paris: UNESCO: Encyclopedia of Life Support Systems. pp. 462–491. ISBN 978-5-8931-7227-0
- "MSNBC article on the U.S. Centers for Disease Control and Prevention report on the prevalence of strength training". Retrieved 2007-02-01

3

Various Athletic Injuries and Health Issues

There are various injuries faced by athletes during their athletic activities. Catastrophic injury, shin splints, tennis elbow, golfer's elbow and anterior cruciate ligament injury are some of the injuries faced by athletes. Athletic training and performance can best be understood in confluence with the major topics listed in the following chapter.

Sports Injury

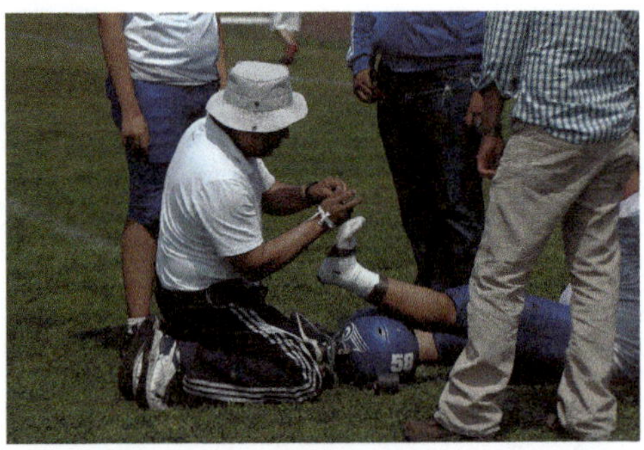

Player getting ankle taped at an American football game in Mexico

Sports injuries are injuries that occur in athletic activities or exercising. In the United States there are about 30 million teenagers and children alone that participate in some form of organized sport. About 3 million avid sports competitors 14 years of age and under experience sports injuries annually, which causes some loss of time of participation in the sport. The leading cause of death involving sports-related injuries, although rare, is brain injuries. When injured the two main systems affected are the nervous and vascular systems. The origins in the body where numbness and tingling occurs upon sports injuries are usually the first signs of the body telling you that the body was impacted. Thus, when an athlete complains of numbness and especially tingling, the key to a diagnosis is to obtain a detailed history of the athlete's acquired symptom perception, determine the effect the injury had on the body and its processes, and then establish the prime treatment method. In the process to determine what exactly happened in the body and the standing effects most medical professionals choose a method of technological medical devices to acquire a credible solution to the site of injury. Prevention helps reduce potential sport injuries. It is important to establish participation in warm-ups, stretching, and exercises that focus on main muscle groups commonly used in the sport of interest. Also, creating an injury prevention program as a team, which includes education on rehydration, nutrition, monitoring team members "at risk", monitoring behavior, skills, and techniques. Season analysis reviews and preseason screenings are also beneficial reviews for preventing player sport injuries. One technique used in the process of preseason screening is the functional movement screen. The functional movement screen can assess movement patterns in athletes in order to find the at risk players. Following various researches about sport injuries shows that levels of anxiety, stress, and depression are elevated. A study in 2010 found that athletes with severe sports injuries would display higher levels of post-traumatic distress and the higher the levels of post-traumatic distress are linked with avoidant coping skills.

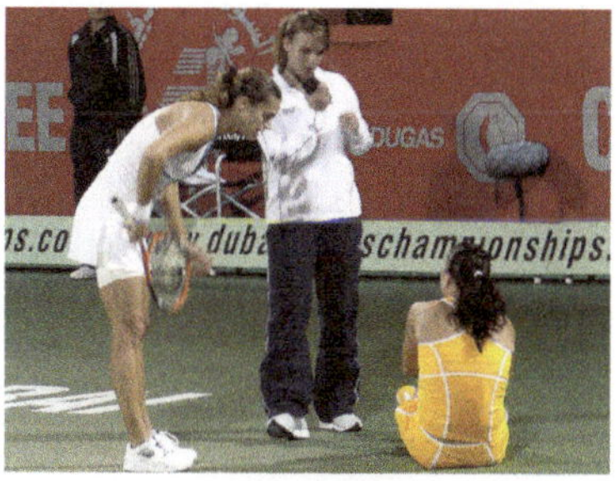

A tennis injury

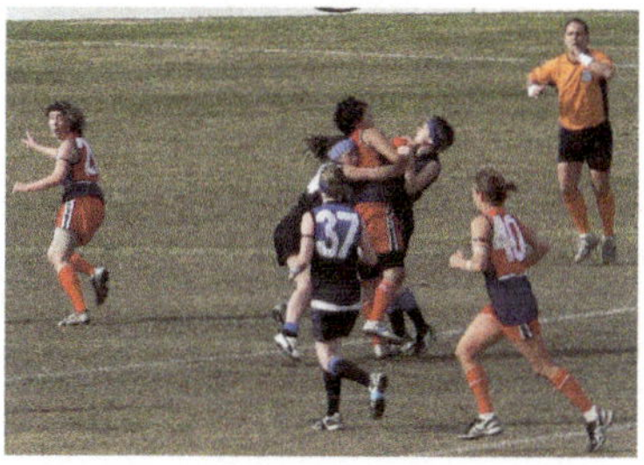

Tackles like this one in women's Australian rules football can cause injuries

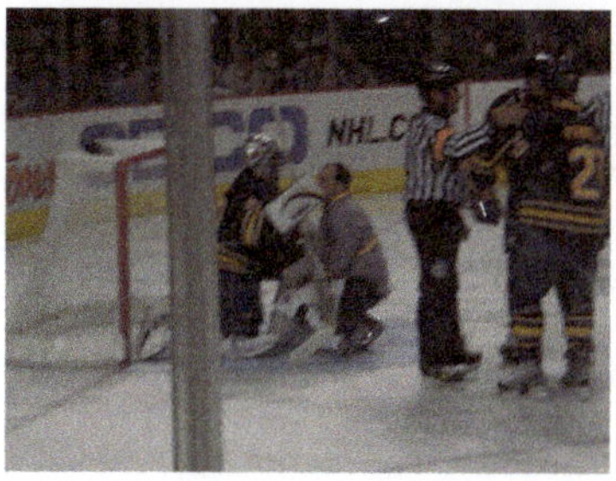

Ryan Miller of the Buffalo Sabres suffers an ankle sprain

Classification

Traumatic injuries account for most injuries in contact sports such as ice hockey, association football, rugby league, rugby union, Australian rules football, Gaelic football and American and Canadian football because of the dynamic and high collision nature of these sports. Collisions with the ground, objects, and other players are common, and unexpected dynamic forces on limbs and joints can cause sports injuries. Nearly two million people every year suffer sports-related injuries and receive treatment in emergency departments. Fatigue is a contributing factor that results in many sport injuries. As an athlete there are times where you may run on low energy leading to the deterioration in technique or form, which results in a slower reaction time, and finally a loss in stability of muscle joints and an injury.

Traumatic injuries can include:

- Contusion or bruise – damage to small blood vessels which causes bleeding within the tissues.
- Strain – trauma to a muscle due to overstretching and tearing of muscle fibers.
- Sprain – an injury in a joint, caused by the ligament being stretched beyond its own capacity.
- Wound – abrasion or puncture of the skin.
- Bone fracture – break(s) in the bone.
- Head injury – concussions or serious brain damage.
- Spinal cord injury – damage to the central nervous system or spine.
- Cramp – a strong muscle contraction that can be very painful lasting in few minutes but massaging the muscles can relieve the pain.

In sports medicine, a catastrophic injury is defined as severe trauma to the human head, spine, or brain.

Concussions in sports became a major issue in the United States in the 2000s, as evidence connected repeated concussions and subconcussive hits with chronic traumatic encephalopathy (CTE) and increased suicide risk. CTE is a progressive degenerative disease of the brain found in people with a history of repetitive brain trauma, including symptomatic concussions as well as subconcussive hits to the head that do not cause symptoms. It is most pronounced in football, and a related ailment (dementia pugilistica) afflicts boxers, but is also seen in other sports, and in females and adolescents. Often, it is has been reported post-mortem.

Overuse and repetitive stress injury problems associated with sports include:

- Runner's knee
- Tennis elbow
- Tendinosis

Some activities have particular risks:

- Bicycle safety
- Gun safety
- Sailing ship accidents
- Skateboarding#Safety

Risk Factors

Intrinsic (Personal) Factors:

- Gender
- Age, weight/body fat, height
- Congenital Irregularities: flat feet, high arch, knocked knees, bow leggedness
- Lack of muscular flexibility, coordination, balance, speed, strength, and endurance
- Malnutrition and lack of sleep

Extrinsic Factors:

- Sports specific and protective equipment: helmet, mouth guard, goggles, shin guards
- Condition of sports setting: maintenance of floor/field and weather environment
- Insufficient pregame warm up, over-training and fatigue

Sports Medicine

Injuries are a common occurrence in professional sports and most teams have a staff of athletic trainers and close connections to the medical community. Many retain team physicians.

Controversy has arisen at times when teams have made decisions that could threaten a player's long-term health for short term gain. Sports medicine is the study and research of injuries in sport in order to prevent or reduce the severity of the injury.

Soft Tissue Injuries

When soft tissue experiences trauma, the dead and damaged cells release chemicals, which initiate an inflammatory response. Inflammation is characterized by pain, localized swelling, heat, redness and a loss of function. Small blood vessels are damaged and opened up, producing bleeding within the tissue. In the body's normal reaction, a small blood clot is formed in order to stop this bleeding and from this clot special cells (called fibroblasts) begin the healing process by laying down scar tissue.

The inflammatory stage is therefore the first phase of healing. However, too much of an inflammatory response in the early stage can mean that the healing process takes longer and a return to activity is delayed. Sports injury treatments are intended to minimize the inflammatory phase of an injury, so that the overall healing process is accelerated. Intrinsic and extrinsic factors are determinant for the healing process.

Prevention

Prevention helps reduce potential sport injuries and provides several benefits. Some benefits include a healthier athlete, longer duration of participation in the sport, potential for better performance, and reduced medical costs. Explaining the benefits to participate in sports injury prevention programs to coaches, team trainers, sports teams, and individual athletes will give them a glimpse at the likelihood for success by having the athletes feeling they are healthy, strong, comfortable, and capable to compete.

Primary, Secondary and Tertiary Prevention

Prevention can be broken up into three broad categories of primary, secondary, and tertiary prevention. Primary prevention involves the avoidance of injury. An example is ankle braces being worn as a team, even those with no history of previous ankle injuries. If primary prevention activities were effective, there would be a lesser chance of injuries occurring in the first place. Secondary prevention involves an early diagnosis and treatment should be acquired once an injury has occurred. The goal of obtaining early diagnosis is to ensure that the injury is receiving proper care and recovering correctly, therefore limiting the concern for other medical problems to stem from the initial traumatic event. Lastly, tertiary prevention is solely focused on the rehabilitation to reduce and correct an existing disability resulting from the traumatic event. An example in the case of an athlete who has obtained an ankle injury the rehabilitation would consist of balance exercises to acquire the strength and mobility back as well as wearing an ankle brace, while gradually returning to the sport.

Season Analysis

It is most essential to establish participation in warm-ups, stretching, and exercises that focus on main muscle groups commonly used in the sport of interest. Participation in these events decreases the chances for getting muscle cramps, torn muscles, and stress fractures. A season analysis is one of the beneficial reviews for preventing player sport injuries. A season analysis is an attempt to identify risks before they occur by reviewing training methods, the competition schedule, traveling, and past injuries. If injuries have occurred in the past, the season analysis reviews the injury and looks for patterns to see if it may be related to a specific training event or competition program. For example, a stress fracture injury on a soccer team or cross country team may be correlated to a simultaneous increase in running and a change in running environment, like a transition from a soft to hard running surface. A season analysis can be documented as team-based results or individual athlete results. Other key program events that have been correlated to injury incidences are changes in training volume, changes in climate locations, selection for playing time in important matches, and poor sleep due to tight chaotic scheduling. It is important for team program directors and staff to implicate testing in order to ensure healthy, competitive, and confident athletes for their upcoming season.

Preseason Screening

Another beneficial review for preventing player sport injuries is preseason screenings. A study found that the highest injury rate during practices across fifteen Division I, II, and III NCAA sports was in the preseason compared to in-season or postseason To prepare an athlete for the wide range of activities needed to partake in their sport pre-participation examinations are regularly completed on hundreds of thousands of athletes each year. It is extremely important that the physical exam is done properly in order to limit the risks of injury and also to diagnose early onsets of a possible injury. Preseason screenings consist of testing the mobility of joints (Ankles, wrists, hips, etc.), testing the stability of joints (knees, neck, etc.), testing the strength and power of muscles, and also testing breathing patterns. The objective of a preseason screening is to clear the athlete for participation and verify that there is no sign of injury or illness, which would represent a potential medical risk to the athlete (and risk of liability to the sports organization). Besides the physical examination and the fluidity of the movements of joints the preseason screenings often takes into account a nutrition aspect as well. It is important to maintain normal iron levels, blood pressure levels, fluid balance, adequate total energy intake, and normal glycogen levels. Nutrition can aid in injury prevention and rehabilitation, if one obtains the body's daily intake needs. Obtaining sufficient amount of calories, carbohydrates, fluids, protein, and vitamins and minerals is important for the overall health of the athlete and limits the risk of possible injuries. Iron deficiency, for example, is found in both male and female athletes; however 60 percent of female college athletes are affected by iron deficiency. There are many factors that can contribute to the loss in iron, like menstruation, gastrointestinal bleeding, inadequate iron intake from the diet, general fatigue, weakness, among others. The consequences of iron deficiency, if not solved, can be an impaired athletic performance and a decline in immune and cognitive function.

Functional Movement Screen

One technique used in the process of preseason screening is the Functional Movement Screen (FMS). Functional movement screening is an assessment used to evaluate movement patterns and asymmetries, which can provide insight into mechanical restrictions and potential risk for injury. Functional movement screening contains seven fundamental movement patterns that require a balance of both mobility and stability. These fundamental movement patterns provide an observable performance of basic locomotor, manipulative, and stabilizing movements. The tests place the individual athlete in extreme positions where weaknesses and imbalances become clear if proper stability and mobility is not functioning correctly. The seven fundamental movement patterns are a deep squat, hurdle step, in-line lunge, shoulder mobility, active straight-leg raise, trunk stability push-up, and rotary stability. For example, the deep squat is a test that challenges total body mechanics. It is used to gauge bilateral, symmetrical, and functional mobility of the hips, knees, and ankles. The dowel held overhead gauges bilateral and symmetrical mobility of the shoulders and the thoracic spine. The ability to perform the deep squat technique requires appropriate pelvic rhythm, closed-kinetic chain dorsiflexion of the ankles, flexion of the knees and hips, extension of the thoracic spine, as well as flexion and abduction of the shoulders. There is a scoring system applied to each movement as follows a score of 3 is given to the athlete if they can perform the movement without any compensations, a score of 2 is given to the athlete if they can perform the movement, but operate on poor mechanics and compensatory patterns to achieve the movement, a score of 1 is given to the athlete if they cannot perform the movement pattern even with compensations, and finally, a 0 is given to the athlete if one has pain during any part of the movement or test. Three of the seven fundamental tests including shoulder mobility, trunk stability push-up, and rotary stability have a clearance scoring associated with them meaning a pass or fail score. If the athlete fails this part of the test a score of 0 is given as the overall score. Once the scoring is complete the athlete and medical professional can review the documentation together and organize a set prevention program to help target and strengthen the areas of weakness in order to limit the risks of possible injuries.

Sport Injury Prevention for Kids

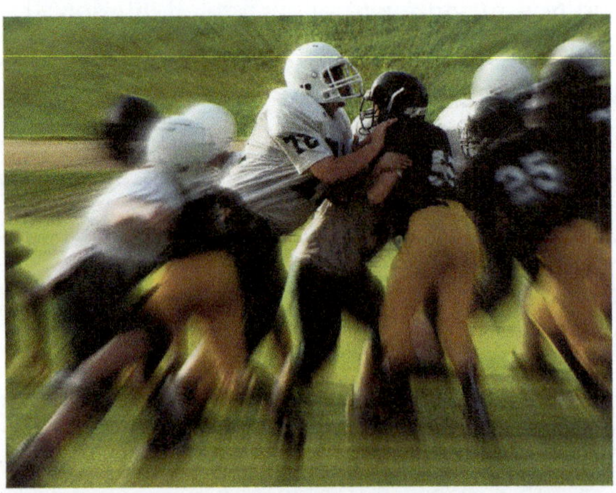

Youths can be easily injured playing contact sports like football.
Proper equipment such as helmets and pads can be helpful in prevention.

There are approximately 8,000 children treated in emergency rooms each day for sports-related injures. It is also estimated that there are around 1.35 million kids suffering from sports-related injuries per year worldwide. This is why children need special attention and care when participating in sports.

According to the Centers for Disease Control and Prevention (CDC), many sports-related injuries are predictable and preventable.

- Kids attending sports clinics tend to know the basic fundamentals of a particular sport. Injury awareness and prevention can also be learned in sports clinics.
- Warming up improves the blood flow in muscles. This brings more nutrients in different parts of the body, therefore bringing more energy throughout.
- Provide children the right equipment on a particular sport like helmets, shin guards, ankle braces, gloves and others to prevent injuries.
- Kids need to have breaks and drink water as well to keep them hydrated.
- Know certain first aid treatment on injuries to apply when there's an unforeseen accident.

Sports Injury Prevalence in College Women

Soccer seems to be the sport leading to most competitive injuries in NCAA female college athletes. Gymnastics, on the other hand, has the highest injury rate overall. For eight of the 13 major sports many injuries acquired during competition require at least seven days recovery before returning to the sport. In general, more females are injured during practice than in competition.

Costs

Interventions targeted at decreasing the incidence of sports injuries can impact health-care costs, as well as family and societal resources. Sports injuries have direct and indirect costs. The direct costs are usually calculated by taking into account the cost of using healthcare resources to prevent, detect and treat injury. There is a need for research about how healthcare is used and the expenses that coincide with it. Included in these expenses are how different injuries may have different prognoses. Indirect costs may be taken into account as well, when an injury prevents an individual from returning to work it may hinder the economic benefit to themselves and others.

Sports-related Emotional Stress

Sport involvement can initiate both physical and mental demands on athletes. From youth little leagues to competing at a professional level, athletes are forced to learn ways to cope with stressors and frustrations that can arise from competition against others. Conducted research shows that levels of anxiety, stress, and depression are elevated following sports injuries. The pressure athletes experience is extensive; branching from coaches, parents, peers, and audiences. It is astonishing how one individual can endure so much pressure and remain so calm and collected. Positive mental motivation however is not experienced all the time. The pressure to win can cause significant emotional stress for an athlete. Many athletes experience the stressor involving winning as being the most important aspect of the match. If the match is not won, many athletes are punished and criticized for the loss, instead of being commended on their effort, sportsmanship, and hard work. After an occurrence of an injury many athletes display self-esteem issues, athletic identity crises, and high levels of post-traumatic distress, which are linked to avoidant coping skills.

Concussions in Sport

Concussions, a type of traumatic brain injury, are a frequent concern for those playing sports, from children and teenagers to professional athletes. Repeated concussions are a known cause of various neurological disorders, most notably chronic traumatic encephalopathy (CTE), which in professional athletes has led to premature retirement, erratic behavior and even suicide. Because concussions cannot be seen on X-rays or CT scans, attempts to prevent concussions have been difficult.

The dangers of repeated concussions have long been known for boxers and wrestlers; a form of CTE common in these two sports, dementia pugilistica (DP), was first described in 1928. An awareness of the risks of concussions in other sports began to grow in the 1990s, and especially in the mid-2000s, in both the medical and the professional sports communities, as a result of studies of the brains of prematurely deceased American football players, who showed extremely high incidences of CTE.

As of 2012, the four major professional sports leagues in the United States and Canada have concussion policies. Sports-related concussions are generally analyzed by athletic training or medical staff on the sidelines using an evaluation tool for cognitive function known as the Sport Concussion Assessment Tool (SCAT), a symptom severity checklist, and a balance test.

Dangers

Concussion symptoms can last for an undetermined amount of time depending on the player and the severity of the concussion. A concussion will affect the way a person's brain works.

There is the potential of post-concussion syndrome, post-concussion syndrome is defined as a set of symptoms that may continue after a concussion is sustained. Post-concussion symptoms can be classified into physical, cognitive, emotional, and sleep symptoms. Physical symptoms include a headache, nausea, and vomiting. Athletes may experience cognitive symptoms that include speaking slowly, difficulty remembering and concentrating. Emotional and sleep symptoms include irritability, sadness, drowsiness, and trouble falling asleep.

Along with the classification of post-concussion symptoms, the symptoms can also be described as immediate and delayed. The immediate symptoms are experienced immediately after a concussion such as: memory loss, disorientation, and poor balance. Delayed symptoms are experienced in the later stages and include sleeping disorders and behavioral changes. Both immediate and delayed symptoms can continue for long periods of time and have a negative impact on recovery. According to research, 20-25% of individuals who have sustained a concussion experienced chronic, delayed symptoms.

Playing through concussion makes people more vulnerable to getting hit again, and that is why most sports have test that trainers will perform to prevent getting hit a second time. A second blow can cause a rare condition known as second-impact syndrome, which can result in severe injury or death. Second-impact syndrome is when an athlete suffers a second head injury before the brain has adequate time to heal in between concussions.

Repeated concussions have been linked to a variety of neurological disorders among athletes, including CTE, Alzheimer's Disease, Parkinsonism and Amyotrophic lateral sclerosis (ALS).

Incidence

It is estimated that as many as 1.6-3.8 million concussions occur in the US per year in competitive sports and recreational activities; this is a rough estimate, since as many as 50% of concussions go unreported. Concussions occur in all sports with the highest incidence in American football, hockey, rugby, soccer, and basketball. In addition to concussions caused by a single severe impact, multiple minor impacts may also cause brain injury.

Injury rate per exposure based on sport in collegiate athletes from 1998 to 2004	
Sport	**Injury rate per 1,000 athletic exposures**
Women's ice hockey	0.91
Men's spring football (American)	0.54
Men's ice hockey	0.41
Women's soccer	0.41
Men's football (American)	0.37
Men's soccer	0.28

Men's wrestling	0.25
Men's lacrosse	0.25
Women's lacrosse	0.25
Women's basketball	0.22
Women's field hockey	0.18
Men's basketball	0.16
Women's gymnastics	0.16
Women's softball	0.14
Women's volleyball	0.09
Men's baseball	0.07
All sports	0.28

Policies

Major League Baseball

Major League Baseball's policy was first started in 2007, and injured players are examined by a team athletic trainer on the field. On March 29, 2011, MLB and the Major League Baseball Players Association announced that they have created various protocols for the league's concussion policy. The new policy includes four primary components:

- All teams are to run baseline neurocognitive testing for all players and umpires using the ImPACT (Immediate Post-Concussion Assessment and Cognitive Testing) system during spring training or after a player signing.
- The SCAT2 (Sport Concussion Assessment Tool, version 2) has been adopted as the official sideline concussion assessment tool of the league, even though various teams have already adopted this tool.
- The establishment of the 7-day disabled list for players with concussions. Players who have been on the list for 14 days are to be transferred to the 15-day list.
- Any player who has been diagnosed with a concussion, regardless of being placed on the disabled list, must have his team submit a return-to-play form to the league's medical director to in order for that player to be cleared to play.

National Basketball Association

The National Basketball Association does not have a policy, and team procedures after concussions vary by team. The NBA has a meeting to educate the players each year about concussions. Players also go through a neurological and cognitive assessment after each season.

During Game 2 of the 2016 NBA Finals on June 5, 2016, Kevin Love was placed in the NBA Concussion Protocol.

National Football League

The National Football League's policy was first started in 2007, and injured players are examined on field by the medical team. The league's policy included the "NFL Sidelines Concussion Exam", which requires players who have taken hits to the head to perform tests concerning concentration, thinking and balance. In 2011, the league introduced an assessment test, which combines a symptoms checklist, a limited neurological examination, a cognitive evaluation, and a balance assessment. For a player to be allowed to return, he must be asymptomatic.

National Hockey League

The National Hockey League's concussion policy began in 1997, and players who sustain concussions are evaluated by a team doctor in a quiet room. In March 2011, the NHL adopted guidelines for the league's concussion policy. Before the adoptions, examinations on the bench for concussions was the minimum requirement, but the new guidelines make it mandatory for players showing concussion like symptoms to be examined by a doctor in the locker room.

"We celebrate the big hit, we don't like the big head hit. There is an important distinction because we celebrate body-checking."

—NHL Commissioner Gary Bettman

League	Year policy first introduced	Year baseline testing occurred	Year current policy became effective	First step after injury	Person who approves/denies player to return	Person who decides player return
NFL	2007	2008	2009	Evaluation by medical team	Medical staff	Medical staff/ Consultant
MLB	2007	2011	2007	Evaluation by an athletic trainer using National Association Guidelines	Medical staff	Head physician/ Medical director
NBA	Never	Never	Never	Depends on team	Depends on team	Depends on team
NHL	1997	1997	2011	Neuropsychological evaluation by team doctor off rink	Team doctor	Team doctor
MLS	2011	2003	2011	Evaluation by medical team	Team physician	Team physician/ Neuropsychologist
NASCAR	2003	2003	2003	Ambulance to infield care center	NASCAR	NASCAR

Concussions in other Sports

American Football

American football causes 250,000 concussions annually, and 20% of high-school football players experience a concussion every year. In 2000, researchers from the Sports Medicine Research Laboratory at the University of North Carolina at Chapel Hill analyzed 17,549 players from 242 different schools. 888 (5.1%) of the players analyzed have at least one concussion a season, and 131 (14.7%) of them have had another concussion the year later. Division III and high-school players have a higher tendency to sustain a concussion than Division II and Division I players. In 2001, the National Football League Players Association partnered with the UNC to determine whether professional football players suffer any health effects after any injuries, although the findings were criticized by the NFL for being unreliable due to being based on self-reporting by the players.

Association Football

Association football— also known as soccer— is a major source of sports-related concussions around the world. Even though 50-80% of injuries in football are directed to the legs, head injuries have been shown to account for between 4 and 22% of football injuries. There is the possibility that heading the ball could damage the head, as the ball can travel at 100 km/hour; although most professional footballers have reported that they experienced head injuries from colliding with other players and the ground. A multi-year study by the University of Colorado published in *JAMA Pediatrics* confirmed that athlete-to-athlete collisions that occur during heading, not impact with the ball itself, is generally the cause for concussion.

A Norwegian study consisting of current and former players of the Norway national football team found out that 3% of the active and 30% of the former players had persistent symptoms of concussions, and that 35% of the active and 32% of that former players had abnormal electroencephalogram (EEG) readings.

During the 2006-07 English Premier League season, Czech goalkeeper Petr Čech suffered from a severe concussion in a match between his club Chelsea and Reading. During the match, Reading midfielder Stephen Hunt hit Čech's head with his right knee, knocking the keeper out. Čech underwent surgery for a depressed skull fracture and was told that he would miss a year of playing football. Čech resumed his goalkeeper duties on January 20, 2007 in a match against Liverpool, now wearing a rugby helmet to protect his weakened skull.

On November 2, 2013 in a match between Tottenham and Everton, Tottenham goal keeper Hugo Lloris sustained a blow to the head by on -coming player Romelu Lukaku's knee. The blow left Lloris knocked out on the ground. Reluctantly manager Andre Villas Boas decided to leave the player on after regaining consciousness and having passed a medical assessment. This broke the rules of the PFA, which state that any player who has lost consciousness must be substituted.

There has been a widespread debate on protective head gear in soccer. Known as a sport associated with intricate footwork, speed, and well-timed passes, soccer also is classified as a high- to moderate-intensity contact/collision sport, with rates of head injury and concussion similar to those seen in football, ice hockey, lacrosse, and rugby. While the benefits of helmets and other head protection are more obvious in the latter sports, the role of headgear in soccer is still unclear.

There are clear rules from FIFA regarding what to do when a player gets a concussion. FIFA's guidelines say that a player who has been knocked unconscious should not play again that day. The rules do however allow for "a transient alteration of conscious level" following a head injury, which says that a player can return to play following assessment by medical staff. The rules also state that a player who is injured with head damage is not to be played for five days.

Among Children and Teenagers

A growing topic is concussions in girls' soccer, predominantly among high-school girls. Studies show that girls are reporting nearly twice as many concussions as boys in the sports that they both play. The number of girls suffering concussions in soccer accounts for the second largest amount of all concussions reported by young athletes. In 2010, more high school soccer players suffered concussions than basketball, baseball, wrestling, and softball players combined, according to the Center for Injury Research and Policy. According to a study in the *JAMA Pediatrics* medical journal, many girls do not getting necessary care and prevention regarding concussions, and 56 percent of players (or their families) reporting concussion symptoms never sought treatment.

According to a 2012 study published by ScienceDirect, soccer has the highest injury rate per athlete-exposure among 7- to 13-year-old children.

Auto Racing

The death of Dale Earnhardt at the 2001 Daytona 500, along with those of Kenny Irwin, Adam Petty and Tony Roper in 2000, and serious injuries sustained by Steve Park in a wreck in September 2001 at Darlington, led to NASCAR establishing numerous policies to assist in driver safety, such as the introduction of the Car of Tomorrow. Drivers were eventually instructed to wear both head and neck restraints, and SAFER barriers have been installed on racetrack walls, with foam-padded supports on each side of the helmet that would allow a driver's head to move in the event of a crash. Despite this, 29 identified concussions occurred between 2004 and 2012.

In 2012, when Dale Earnhardt, Jr. suffered a concussion after being involved in a crash at the end of the Good Sam Roadside Assistance 500 at Talladega, NASCAR expressed consideration in adding baseline testing to its concussion policies. NASCAR was one of few motorsport organizations that do not have baseline testing, though that ended in 2014, as baseline testing started being performed at the start of the seasons.

Basketball

In the 2005 high school basketball year, 3.6% of reported injuries were concussions, with 30.5% of concussions occurring during rebounds. Incidence rates for concussions in NCAA men's basketball is lower than NCAA women's basketball, at 0.16 concussion per 1,000 athletes compared to 0.22 per 1,000 athletes respectively. The difference is found mainly in competition activity compared to practice.

Boxing

Despite boxing's violent nature, a National Safety Council report in 1996 ranked amateur boxing as the safest contact sport in America. However, concussions are one of the most serious injuries that can occur from boxing, and in an 80-year span from 1918 to 1998, there were 659 boxers who died from brain injury. Incidence rates for concussion in boxing may frequently be miscalculated due to the fact that concussions do not always result from a knockout blow.

Gymnastics

As many skills as gymnastics involve flipping or a blind landing, incidence of head injury increases. A 15 year study found an incidence of 1.7% for concussion and closed head injury for high school gymnasts.

Ice Hockey

Ice hockey has also been known to have concussions inflict numerous players. Because of this, the NHL made hockey helmets mandatory in the 1979–80 NHL season. According to a data release by the National Academy of Neuropsychology's Sports Concussion Symposium, from 2006 to 2011, 765 NHL players were diagnosed with a concussion. At the Mayo Clinic Sports Medicine Center Ice Hockey Summit: Action on Concussion conference in 2010, a panel made a recommendation that blows to the head are to be prohibited, and to outlaw body checking by 11- and 12-year-olds. For the 2010–11 NHL season, the NHL prohibited blindside hits to the head, but did not ban hits to the face. The conference also urged the NHL and its minor entities to join the International Ice Hockey Federation, the NCAA and the Ontario Hockey League in banning any contact to the head.

The NHL has been criticized for allowing team doctors to determine whether an injured player can return to the ice, instead of independent doctors.

Rugby Union

Concussions are also a significant factor in rugby union, another full-contact sport. In 2011, the sport's world governing body, World Rugby (then known as the International Rugby Board, or IRB), issued a highly detailed policy for dealing with injured players with suspected concussions. Under the policy, a player suffering from a suspected concussion is not allowed to return to play in that game. Players are not cleared to play after the injury for a minimum of 21 days, unless they are being supervised in their recovery by a medical practitioner. Even when medical advice is present, players must complete a multi-step monitoring process before being cleared to play again; this process requires a minimum of six days. In 2012, the IRB modified the policy, instituting a Pitchside Suspected Concussion Assessment (PSCA), under which players suspected of having suffered concussions are to leave the field for 5 minutes while doctors assess their condition via a series of questions. Players who pass the PSCA are allowed to return to play.

However, an incident during the third Test of the 2013 Lions tour of Australia led to criticism of the current protocols. During that match, Australian George Smith clashed heads with the Lions' Richard Hibbard and was sent to pitchside. According to ESPN's UK channel, "despite looking dazed and confused, Smith passed the PSCA and was back on the field minutes later."

In 2013, former Scotland international Rory Lamont charged that the current concussion protocols can easily be manipulated. A key part of the current protocols is the "Cogsport" test (also known as COG), a computer-based test of cognitive function. Each player undergoes the test before the start of a new season, and is then tested again on it after a head injury, and the results compared, to determine possible impairment. According to Lamont, some players deliberately do poorly on the pre-season test, so that they will be more likely to match or beat their previous results during play.

Lamont was also critical of the PSCA, noting:

> "The problem with the PSCA is a concussed player can pass the assessment. I know from first hand experience it can be quite ineffective in deciding if a player is concussed. It is argued that allowing the five-minutes assessment is better than zero minutes but it is not as clear cut as one might hope. Concussion symptoms regularly take 10 minutes or longer to actually present. Consequently the five-minute PSCA may be giving concussed players a license to return to the field."

The Concussion bin was replaced by the head bin in 2012 with the players assessment taking 10 minutes. If concussed the player must then recover by first returning to general activities in life, then progressing back to playing. Returning to play, the player must follow the Graduated Return to Play (GRTP) protocol, by having clearance from a medical professional, and no symptoms of concussion.

Female Sports

Numerous reports have indicated that female athletes suffer more concussions than male athletes. A December 2008 report states that 29,167 female high school soccer players in the United States suffered from concussions in 2005, compared to 20,929 male players. In high school basketball, 12,923 girls suffered from concussions while only 3,823 boys did. Girls also sustained more concussions in softball, compared to boys in baseball. Female athletes also had longer recovery times than males, and also had lower scores on visual memory tests. Girls also have longer recovery times for concussions, which may be due to a greater rate of blood flow in the brain.

Women's ice hockey was reported as one of the most dangerous sports in the NCAA, with a concussion rate of 2.72 per 1,000 player hours. Even though men's ice hockey allows body checking, while women's ice hockey does not, the rate of concussions for men is 46% lower, at 1.47 per 1,000 player hours. College football also has lower concussion rates than women's hockey, with a rate of 2.34 per 1,000.

Women's basketball is one of the women's sports with the highest risks of getting a concussion. Women have a greater risk of getting a concussion by dribbling/ball handling rather than defending. Also it was found that female college basketball players typically receive concussions during games rather than practices.

Prevention Efforts and Technology

There have been numerous attempts at preventing concussions, such as the establishment of the PACE (Protecting Athletes Through Concussion Education) program, which works with the imPACT system, which is currently used by every NFL and some NHL teams. In 2008, the Arena Football League tested an impact monitor created by Schutt Sports called the "Shockometer", which is a triangular device attached to the back of football helmets that has a light on the device that turns red when a concussion occurs. Riddell has also created the Head Impact Telemetry System (HITS) and Sideline Response System (SRS) to record the frequency and severity of player hits during practices and games. On every helmet with the system, MX Encoders are implemented, which can automatically record every hit. Eight NFL teams had originally planned to use the system in the 2010 season, but the NFL Players Association ultimately blocked its use. Other impact-detection devices include CheckLight, by Reebok and MC10., and the online test providers ImPACT Test, BrainCheck, and XLNTbrain which establish cognitive function baselines against which the athlete is monitored over time. The CCAT online tool developed by Axon Sports is another test to assist doctors in assessing concussion.

Media Coverage

In 2012, film producer Steve James created the documentary film *Head Games*, interviewing former NHL player Keith Primeau, and the parents of Owen Thomas, who hanged himself after sustaining brain damage during his football career at Penn. The documentary also interviewed former athletes Christopher Nowinski, Cindy Parlow, and *New York Times* reporter Alan Schwarz, among other athletes, journalists, and medical researchers.

League of Denial was a 2013 book by sports reporters Mark Fainaru-Wada and Steve Fainaru about concussions within the NFL. The American documentary series *Frontline* covered the topic in two episodes, one based on the book and also called "League of Denial", and the other called "Football High" Political sports journalist Dave Zirin has also covered the topic in detail.

Running Injuries

Running is a form of exercise and described as the one of the world's most accessible sport. However, its high-impact nature can lead to injury. Approximately 50% of runners are affected by some form of running injuries or running-related injuries (RRI) annually, and some estimates suggest an even higher frequency. The frequency of various RRI depend on the type of running, as runners vary significantly in factors such as speed and mileage. RRI can be both acute and chronic. Many of the common injuries that plague runners are chronic, developing over a longer period of time, as opposed to injury caused by sudden trauma, such as strains. These are often the result of overuse. Common overuse injuries include stress fractures, Achilles tendinitis, Iliotibial band syndrome, Patellofemoral pain (runners knee), and plantar fasciitis.

Proper running form is important in injury prevention. A major aspect of running form is foot strike pattern. The way in which the foot makes contact with the ground determines how the force of the impact is distributed throughout the body. Different types of modern running shoes are created to manipulate foot strike pattern in an effort to reduce the risk of injury. In recent years, barefoot running has increased in popularity in many western countries, because of claims that it reduces the risk of injury. However, this is has not been proven and is still debated.

Overuse Injuries

Causes and Prevention

In general, overuse injuries are the result of repetitive impact between the foot and the ground. With improper running form, the force of the impact can be distributed abnormally throughout the feet and legs. Running form tends to worsen with fatigue. When moving at a constant pace, a symmetrical gait is considered to be normal. Asymmetry is considered to be a risk factor for injury. One study attempted to quantify the change in running form between a rested and fatigued state by measuring asymmetrical running gait in the lower limbs. The results showed that "knee internal rotation and knee stiffness became more asymmetrical with fatigue, increasing by 14% and 5.3%, respectively". These findings suggest that focusing on proper running form, particularly when fatigued, could reduce the risk of running related injuries. Running in worn out shoes may also increase the risk of injury and altering the footwear might be helpful. These injuries can also arise due to a sudden increase in the intensity or amount of exercise.

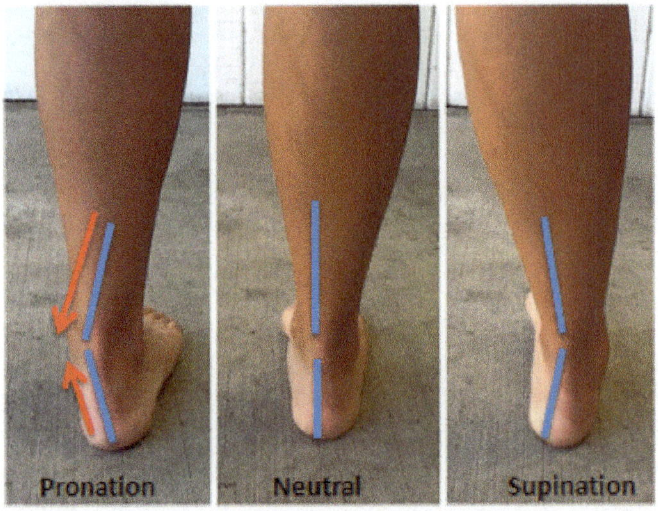

Pronation neutral and supination placements of the right ankle.
The ankle and foot naturally pronate and supinate by about 5 degrees while walking or running. The red arrows indicate excessive pronation.

Achilles Tendinitis

Achilles tendinitis is the inflammation of the Achilles tendon, resulting in pain along the back of the leg near the heel. There are two types of Achilles tendinitis, insertional and noninsertional. Noninsertional Achilles tendinitis is the type that more commonly affects runners. In this case, inflammation is occurring in the middle portion of the tendon, whereas insertional Achilles tendinitis is inflammation located where the tendon connects (inserts) to the heel bone. Having tight calf muscles may also increase the risk of Achilles tendinitis. Stretching the calves before starting heavy exercise may help relieve tightness in the muscles.

Patellofemoral Pain Syndrome

Patellofemoral pain syndrome is associated with pain in the knee and around the patella. It is sometimes referred to as runner's knee, but this term is used for other overuse injuries that involve knee pain as well. It can be caused by a single incident, but is often the result of overuse or a sudden icrease in physical activity.

Iliotibial Band Syndrome

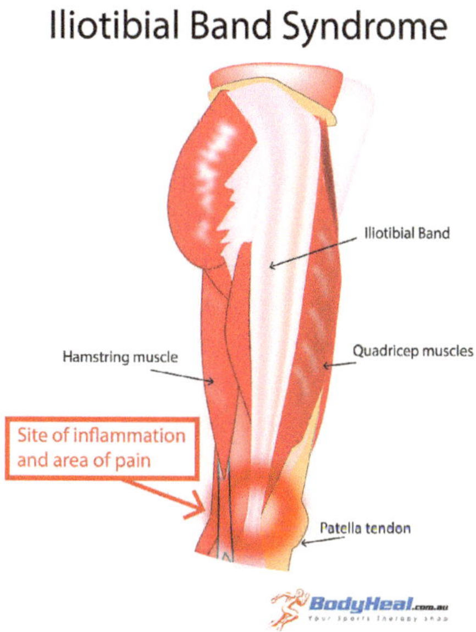

Diagram indicating the location of the iliotibial band and pain associated with iliotibial band syndrome

Iliotibial band syndrome is defined as inflammation of the iliotibial band on the outside of the knee. This inflammation occurs a result of the iliotibial band and the outside of the knee join rubbing together. The resulting pain typically is initially mild and worsens if running continues. Recurrence is a common issue with iliotibial band syndrome, as pain goes away with a period of rest, but symptoms can easily come back as the runner returns to training. During recovery, the muscles on the outside of the hip can be stretched to reduce tightness in the band.

Footwear

Traditional Running Shoes

So called 'traditional' running shoes are designed to give more support and cushion the landing to reduce the effects of impact. They allow for more comfortable running on hard surfaces such as asphalt and also protect the foot when stepping on rocks or other potentially sharp objects. However, the cushioning provided in traditional running shoes is thought to encourage a foot strike pattern, where the heel lands first. Heel striking generates a relatively large amount of impact force that can put different parts of the lower extremities under excessive stress.

Barefoot Running

Barefoot running has been promoted as one method of reducing the risk of running related injuries. Barefoot running is thought to improve running form by encouraging forefoot striking. The collision of the forefoot with the ground generates a significantly smaller impact force in comparison to striking heel first. However, barefoot running leaves the foot unprotected from stepping on sharp objects. Although running barefoot may reduce the risk of running related injuries, it is important to take time while switching from running with shoes.

Beginning to run barefoot without reducing intensity or mileage of training can actually cause muscle or tendon injury. Changing one's style of running shoe or switching to barefoot running will most likely alter the foot strike pattern, meaning that the force of impact will be absorbed differently. Injuries are more likely to occur in novice barefoot runners. This may be a result of not yet having fully adapted to a new style of running, and therefore running with inconsistent technique. To measure this, a study was conducted involving runners who habitually run with a rearfoot strike while wearing shoes. Of the runners involved in the study, 32% used a heel strike pattern in initial attempts at running barefoot. Running barefoot while heel striking leads to increased muscle activation and impact accelerations. The findings suggest that an inconsistency in running technique among novice barefoot runners may put them at a higher risk of injury in comparison to running with shoes.

Under some hypotheses, humans and their recent evolutionary ancestors may have needed to be able to run long distances in order to survive, and therefore natural selection would have favored traits that improve humans ability to run for long periods of time.

Endurance Running Hypothesis

According to the endurance running hypothesis, long distance running has been suggested to have played significant role in the lifestyle and evolution of early hominins. Before developing more advance hunting tools such as the bow and arrow, are thought to have used endurance running for scavenging and hunting. Persistence hunting is "a form of pursuit hunting in which [the hunter uses] endurance running during the midday heat to drive [prey] into hyperthermia and exhaustion so they can easily be killed". Unlike many medium-to-large mammals that use panting as a form of evaporative cooling, hominins rely on sweating, allowing evaporation to occur on a much larger surface area. In this way, sweating results in better thermoregulation that allows the hominin to outlast the prey during the chase. This is one potential explanation for the loss of most body hair in humans. Those individuals with less body hair would be able to better thermoregulate while running to avoid overheating. For this species to exist under the endurance running hypothesis, running most likely did not result in the frequency of injuries that it does today, because such an injury to early hominins likely lead to starvation. This example would imply that recent ancestors of humans experienced selective pressure to adapt to barefoot running.

Minimalist Footwear

Minimalist shoes are an alternative option that can be seen as an intermediate between running barefoot or with traditional running shoes, as they lack the high cushioned heels of traditional running shoes. These shoes are also designed to encourage forefoot striking. One study observed the redistribution of mechanical work with fast speed running in minimalist shoes compared to conventional shoes in 26 trained runners. The results showed that running at a fast pace in minimalist shoes caused a statistically significant redistribution of work from the knee to the ankle joint. Therefore, switching to a minimalist running shoe may be beneficial in preventing recurrence for runners who have experienced a knee injury in the past. However, the switch could also increase the risk of ankle and calf injuries. As with to barefoot running, runners who chose to switch to minimalist shoes should not start out at full training intensity.

Iliotibial band syndrome (ITBS or ITBFS, for iliotibial band friction syndrome) is a common injury to the knee, generally associated with running, cycling, hiking or weight-lifting (especially squats).

Definition

Iliotibial band syndrome is one of the leading causes of lateral knee pain in runners. The iliotibial band is a thick band of fascia on the lateral aspect of the knee, extending from the outside of the pelvis, over the hip and knee, and inserting just below the knee. The band is crucial to stabilizing the knee during running, as it moves from behind the femur to the front of the femur during activity. The continual rubbing of the band over the lateral femoral epicondyle, combined with the repeated flexion and extension of the knee during running may cause the area to become inflamed.

Signs and Symptoms

ITBS symptoms range from a stinging sensation just above the knee joint, to swelling or thickening of the tissue in the area where the band moves over the femur. The stinging sensation just above the knee joint is felt on the outside of the knee or along the entire length of the iliotibial band. Pain may not occur immediately during activity, but may intensify over time. Pain is most commonly felt when the foot strikes the ground, and pain might persist after activity. Pain may also be present above and below the knee, where the ITB attaches to the tibia. It will also hurt if you twist your knee to turn a corner.

Causes

ITBS can result from one or more of the following: training habits, anatomical abnormalities, or muscular imbalances:

Training habits	Abnormalities in leg/feet anatomy
• Spending long periods of time/regularly sitting in lotus posture in yoga. Esp beginners forcing the feet onto the top of the thighs • Consistently running on a horizontally banked surface (such as the shoulder of a road or an indoor track) on which the downhill leg is bent slightly inward, causing extreme stretching of the band against the femur • Inadequate warm-up or cool-down • Excessive up-hill and down-hill running • Positioning the feet "toed-in" to an excessive angle when cycling • Running up and down stairs • Hiking long distances • Rowing • Breaststroke • Treading water	• High or low arches • Supination of the foot • Excessive lower-leg rotation due to over-pronation • Excessive foot-strike force • Uneven leg lengths • Bowlegs or tightness about the iliotibial band. **Muscle imbalance** • Weak hip abductor muscles • Weak/non-firing multifidus muscle • Uneven left-right stretching of the band, which could be caused by habits such as sitting cross-legged

Treatment

While ITBS pain can be acute, the iliotibial band can be rested, iced, compressed and elevated (RICE) to reduce pain and inflammation, followed by stretching. Massage therapy, and many of its modalities, can offer relief if symptoms arise.

Catastrophic Injury

A catastrophic injury is a severe injury to the spine, spinal cord, or brain, and may also include skull or spinal fractures. This is a subset of the definition for the legal term *catastrophic injury*, which is based on the definition used by the American Medical Association.

The National Center for Catastrophic Sport Injury Research in the United States classifies catastrophic injuries based on the three outcomes associated with them: fatality, those causing permanent severe functional disability, and those causing severe head or neck trauma with no permanent disability. A fatal injury may be a direct result of trauma sustained during an activity, or may occur indirectly. Indirect nonfatal catastrophic injury may occur as a result of systemic failure from exertion during an activity, such as from cardiovascular conditions, heat illness, exertional hyponatremia, or dehydration, or a complication to a nonfatal injury. Indirect fatalities are usually caused by cardiovascular conditions, such as hypertrophic cardiomyopathy and coronary artery disease.

Fatal injury may reveal an unknown "underlying anatomical or physiological abnormality". Individuals with certain anatomical anomalies should not participate in some activities. For example, contact sports are contraindicated for individuals with an anomalous odontoid process, as any violent impact may result in a catastrophic injury. This is because a malformed odontoid process may lead to instability between the atlas and axis (the C1 and C2 cervical vertebrae). Those with atlanto-occipital fusion should also avoid contact sports.

By Activity

Participation in any sport or recreational activity may result in a catastrophic sports injury, particularly if unsupervised or if engaged with little or no protection. Direct fatalities in sport are rare, as most sport fatalities are indirect and associated with non-sport cardiovascular problems.

In the United States, American football has the greatest incidence of catastrophic injury per population, whereas cheerleading is associated with the greatest incidence of direct catastrophic injury at both the interscholastic and intercollegiate levels.

Cervical spine trauma is most common in sports and activities involving contact and collision, particularly American football, rugby, ice hockey, gymnastics, skiing, wrestling, and diving. A 2005 report by the National Center for Catastrophic Sport Injury Research in the United States stated that sports requiring attention for potential catastrophic injuries are American football, ice hockey, baseball, wrestling, gymnastics, and track and field.

The incidence of catastrophic injury is four times higher in college than in high school in the United States. Sport accounts for between 5% and 10% of all cervical spine and spinal cord injuries in the United States, and 15% in Australia. The incidence of catastrophic injury for all sports is low, less than 0.5 per 100,000 participants.

A study in the province of Ontario in Canada based on epidemiological data from 1986, 1989, 1992, and 1995 states that the greatest incidence of catastrophic injuries occurred in snowmobiling, cycling, ice hockey, and skiing. Of the 2,154 reported catastrophic injuries, 1,756 were sustained by males and 368 by females. The only activity in the study in which female casualties outnumbered males was equestrianism. The study also stated that field and floor sports had a relatively low incidence of catastrophic injury, and that July had the highest incidence of injury. Drowning was the cause of 357 fatalities, and there were 640 head and 433 spine injuries.

The study found 79.2% of the injuries were preventable; from over 1,500 responses, 346 involved alcohol consumption, and 1,236 were not supervised. Most alcohol-related injuries were sustained in snowmobiling (124), fishing (41), diving (40), boating excluding canoeing (31), swimming (31), riding an all-terrain vehicle (24), and cycling (23). Other studies have concluded that alcohol consumption is a common risk factor "associated with all types of exposure" (that is, activities) for traumatic brain injury.

Classification of Sports by Contact

The American Academy of Pediatrics has classified sports based on the likelihood of collision and contact. It recommends against participation in boxing.

Those classified as *contact and collision* sports include basketball, boxing, diving, field hockey, football, ice hockey, lacrosse, martial arts, rodeo, rugby, ski jumping, soccer, team handball, water polo, and wrestling.

Those classified as *limited contact* include baseball, bicycling, cheerleading, whitewater canoeing and kayaking, fencing, floor hockey, flag football, gymnastics, handball, horseback riding, racquetball, skating (ice skating, inline skating, roller skating), skiing (cross-country skiing, downhill skiing, water skiing), skateboarding, snowboarding, softball, squash, ultimate frisbee, volleyball, and windsurfing or surfing, and the track and field events high jump and pole vaulting.

Sports classified as *non-contact* include archery, badminton, body building, bowling, flat-water canoeing and kayaking, curling, dancing, golf, orienteering, power lifting, race walking, riflery, rope jumping, rowing, running, sailing, scuba diving, swimming, table tennis, tennis, weightlifting and weight training, the track and field events discus, javelin, and shot put and all track events.

American Football

From 1945 to 2005, there were 497 fatalities, of which 69% were a result of brain injury and 16% from spinal cord injury. Today, the most common catastrophic injury in American football is cervical spinal cord injury, which is also the "second leading cause of death attributable to football". The 84% reduction in head injuries and 74% reduction in fatalities is directly attributable to the implementation of NOCSAE standards for football helmets and rule changes for tackling.

Football has the highest incidence of cervical spinal cord injuries in the United States per population. From 1977 to 2001, the incidence of cervical spinal cord injury amongst high school, college, and professional participants was 0.52, 1.55, and 14 per 100,000 participants, respectively.

From 1982 to 1988, 75% of direct fatalities and 40% of indirect fatalities in college sports were associated with football; for high school athletes, the rates were 75% and 33%, respectively. Indirect fatalities were usually caused by cardiac failure or heat exhaustion. Indirect fatalities in high school and college football have been attributed to heat stroke, heart-related conditions, viral meningitis, and even lightning strikes.

The most common mechanism for catastrophic cervical spinal cord injury in American football is axial loading or compression resultant from spear tackling, in which a player uses the crown of the helmet as the initial point of contact for striking another player. This form of tackling was banned in 1976 for high school and college football, resulting in a significant reduction in catastrophic injuries of this type. For example, incidence of quadriplegia decreased from 2.24 and 10.66 per 100,000 participants in high school and college football in 1976, to 1.30 and 2.66 per 100,000 participants in 1977. Since 1977, about 67% of all catastrophic injuries in football were the result of a player making a tackle.

In the paper *Catastrophic Football Injuries: 1977-1998* published in 2000 by the journal *Neurosurgery*, Robert Cantu and Frederick Mueller recommend that "players should use the shoulder for blocking and tackling" instead of "using the head as a battering ram". The purpose of rules against spearing, ramming, and butting is to protect both the tackler and the opponent from head trauma or catastrophic injury. Mueller also suggests that coaches remove players from a game if they exhibit symptoms of concussion, such as dizziness, headaches, nausea, or sensitivity to light.

Baseball

Baseball has a high incidence of catastrophic injury, the most common being cranial injuries usually sustained during a collision between a baserunner diving head first and a fielder, resulting in an axial compression injury to the baserunner. Other causes included collisions, such as between a catcher and baserunner, or being struck by a pitched or thrown ball.

Canoeing

In the Ontario study, all catastrophic injuries recorded for recreational canoeing were fatal, and accounted for 4.3% of all sport and recreation fatalities in the province. Of the 27 cases, 24 fatalities resulted from drowning, and the others from cerebral contusions, cerebral lacerations, and skull fractures. Canoeing drowning fatalities are "often correlated with alcohol consumption", as it increases the probability of submersion and decreases the probability of recovery from submersion. They are often associated with young males inexperienced in canoeing.

Cheerleading

The primary cause of increased incidence of catastrophic injuries to cheerleaders is the "evolution of cheerleading to a gymnastic-like activity". It is the leading cause of catastrophic injuries to females, representing over 65% of the catastrophic injuries occurring in high school and college female athletes in the United States.

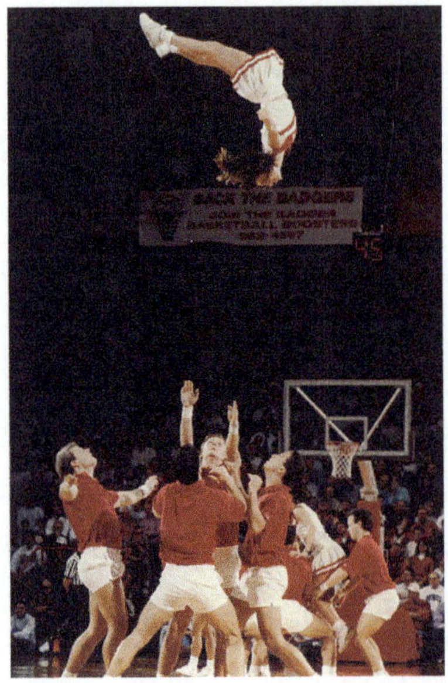

Cheerleading tosses and vaults, particularly when performed over a hard surface, are a high-risk activity

High-risk activities include the construction of pyramids, which result in several catastrophic injuries each year, the 'basket toss', and tumbling, all of which are usually performed over hard surfaces. Cheerleader pyramids are banned in Minnesota and North Dakota.

Other causes include inadequate supervision, poorly trained coaches, and the equipment used.

Fishing

In the Ontario study, fishing resulted in 126 catastrophic injuries, of which 117 were fatal, 110 from drowning. Of these, 119 events were associated with males, of which 112 were fatalities. Fishing had the highest rate of catastrophic injuries to all injuries for any activity in Ontario, as 2.54% of all fishing injuries were catastrophic.

Catastrophic injuries in fishing may be related to equipment, fish, alcohol, or the environment. Equipment issues generally involve penetrative injuries from the use of hooks and harpoons, but may also be caused by the fishing rod, lure, sinker, or bait. Fish-related injuries result from mishandling, poisoning, and contamination from consumption. Environmental causes may include overexposure to solar radiation, lightning strikes, hypothermia during ice fishing, snakebites, and viral infection spread by mosquitoes.

Gymnastics

Gymnastics has a relatively low incidence of catastrophic injury, that is the number of catastrophic injuries with respect to the number of participants. In the United States from 1982 to 2007, nineteen catastrophic injuries were reported from 147 million high school and 8 million college participants.

Club-level injury surveillance data in Australia indicate no catastrophic injury to elite participants from 1983 to 1993. Elite gymnast catastrophic injuries to the spinal cord have been recorded in China, Japan, and the United States, the most notable being to Sang Lan and Julissa Gomez. There is an "absence of research reporting rate data" for catastrophic injury to club-level gymnasts in the United States.

Ice Hockey

The most common catastrophic injury occurring in ice hockey is cervical spinal cord injury, which most often occur at C5, C6, or C7. The most common cause is checking from behind. Such checking was banned from hockey in 1985, which has resulted in a decreased incidence of catastrophic spinal injuries and a reduction of head and neck injuries.

Increased standards for hockey helmets and the requirement that they be worn in competitive play has resulted in a decrease of serious head injury and fatalities. Although full facial protection (helmet with cage) did not reduce the incidence of catastrophic injuries or concussion compared to a standard helmet, it reduced the incidence of facial injuries and lacerations.

Porting

Porters who carry loads on their heads are subjected to axial strains that exacerbate degenerative change in the cervical spine, and has an etiological role in spondylosis.

In a 1968 study, Laurence Levy recorded six catastrophic injuries to porters at Harare Central Hospital in Harare, Zimbabwe. Of these, one died instantaneously, and five became quadriplegic, one as a result of a herniated intervertebral disc and four from fractures or fracture-dislocations.

Rugby

For rugby union, the incidence of catastrophic injury from 1952 to 2005 in England was 0.84 per 100,000 per year. In all other countries, from 1970 to 2007 the incidence was 4.6 per 100,000 per year. For rugby league, it was 2 per 100,000 per year. In rugby union in France, the incidence of catastrophic cervical spine injuries decreased from 2.1 per 100,000 in the 1996–1997 season to 1.4 per 100,000 in the 2005–2006 season, which has been attributed to rule changes regarding the scrum.

The most common causes are the scrum, the ruck or maul, and the tackle. Research from Australia states that injury prevention in youth rugby should focus on the scrum and the tackle, and that risk factors are level of play (age group) and player position. It also indicated that "neck injuries in the scrum and to the front row are of great concern".

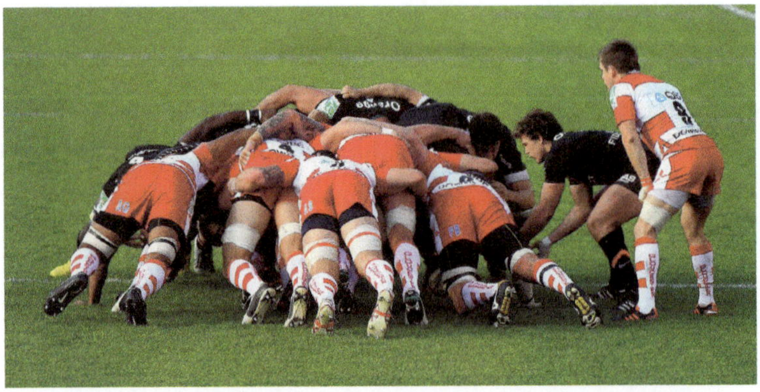

Rugby scrums are high-risk activities for catastrophic injury

The use of a scrum cap or other padded headgear does not reduce the incidence of concussion or other head or neck trauma.

Skiing and Snowboarding

In a survey of scientific literature from 1990 to 2004, 24 studies covering 10 countries indicated an increasing incidence of traumatic brain injury (TBI) and spinal cord injury amongst alpine skiers and snowboarders. The most common cause of death is head injuries, which can be mitigated by 22–60% by the use of helmets. The increased incidence coincides "with the development and acceptance of acrobatic and high-speed activities".

Most deaths are attributed to massive head, neck, or thoracoabdominal injury, of which TBI accounted for between 50% and 88% and spinal cord injury between 1% and 13%. Ski fatalities occur between 0.050 and 0.196 per 100,000 participants. Head injuries represent 28.0% of all injuries in skiers and 33.5% for snowboarders.

Snowmobiling

In the Ontario study, snowmobiling had the highest incidence and prevalence of recreational catastrophic injuries of any activity (290 incidents, 120 fatalities). It had the second-highest incidence of catastrophic injury per participant (88.2 per 100,000), the greatest incidence per 100,000 population (0.706), and the greatest incidence of fatality per 100,000 population (0.292). It was also the activity in which alcohol consumption was most prevalent in catastrophic events (124), representing more than one third of all events for which alcohol was a factor. Other contributing factors include "poor lighting, young age and inappropriate terrain".

Track and Field

The majority of track and field-related fatalities in the United States is associated with pole vaulting. Other fatalities and catastrophic injuries in track and field occur by a participant or bystander being struck by a discus, shot put, or javelin.

Water Sports

Most catastrophic injuries related to diving and swimming in the United States occur when an individual dives into shallow water. It is the cause of 2.6% of all cervical spine injury admissions, and are chiefly sustained by recreational divers. The most common cause is diving into shallow water, inexperience, inadequate supervision, and alcohol consumption.

Catastrophic swimming injuries in the Ontario study were four times as prevalent in males than females. The incidence of catastrophic injury in competitive swimming is very low, and almost all such injuries occur in recreational and non-competitive swimming.

Wrestling

From 1981 until 1999 in the United States, 35 catastrophic injuries related to wrestling were reported, one in college and the others in high school, an incidence of 1 per 10,000 per year. They were caused by three positions: defensive position during takedown (74%), down position (23%), and lying position (3%). Most occurred in the lower weight classes, and 80% were incurred during a match. In Iran from 1998 to 2005, the incidence of catastrophic injury was 1.99 per 100,000 participants per year.

Most injuries were cervical fracture or major cervical ligament injuries. One of the athletes died, one third became tetraplegic, one paraplegic, and six others suffered residual neurologic deficit.

Catastrophic wrestling injuries are preventable, and associated risk factors include incorrectly performing a manouevre, lack of supervision by the coach, and inappropriate injury management.

Other Activities

In the United Kingdom, the incidence of catastrophic injury per year for work-related situations is 0.9 per 100,000. The incidence is highest in agriculture (6.0 per 100,000) and construction (6.0 per 100,000), and lowest in the service sector (0.4).

The incidence is 3.7 per 100,000 for pedestrians, 2.9 per 100,000 for automobile occupants, and 190 per 100,000 for motorcyclists.

Vehicular accidents account for 43% of catastrophic spinal injury in the United States and 45% in Australia.

In the Ontario study, recreational catastrophic injuries were most prevalent in snowmobiling (290 incidents, 120 fatalities), bicycling (289 incidents, 67 fatalities), fishing (126 incidents, 117 fatalities), boating (excluding canoeing, 112 incidents, 72 fatalities), diving (105 incidents, 5 fatalities) and swimming (100 incidents, 86 fatalities). The greatest incidence per participant was recorded for diving (511.0 per 100,000), snowmobiling (88.2 per 100,000), parachuting (62.9 per 100,000), tobogganing or sledding (37.7 per 100,000), hang gliding (29.4 per 100,000), water polo (24.5 per 100,000), scuba diving (12.2 per 100,000), hunting (12.2 per 100,000), horseback riding (11.6 per 100,000), archery (11.1 per 100,000), and fishing (11.0 per 100,000). The greatest incidence per 100,000 population were recorded for snowmobiling (0.706), cycling (0.701), ice hockey (0.462), fishing (0.307), boating excluding canoeing (0.273), diving (0.256), swimming (0.243) and baseball (0.217). The greatest incidence of fatality per 100,000 population were recorded for snowmobiling (0.292), fishing (0.285), swimming (0.200), boating excluding canoeing (0.175), cycling (0.163), canoeing (0.066), riding an all-terrain vehicle (0.039), hunting (0.037), and horseback riding (0.024). Catastrophic cycling injuries were most prevalent in cities, particularly Toronto (64), Ottawa (21), and London (7). Drowning represented more than half of sport and recreation fatalities in the Ontario study.

In the United States, the Consumer Product Safety Commission (CPSC) recorded nearly 1,000 fatalities between 1967 and 1987 as a result of riding an all-terrain vehicle, more than half of which were individuals less than 16 years old. This led to a filing of an action per the Consumer Product Safety Act in 1987, which effectively ended the sale of three-wheeled ATVs. Since then, 35% of deaths were individuals less than 16 years old. The American Academy of Pediatrics and CPSC recommend that individuals less than 16 years old should not ride ATVs.

Effects and Management

The types of acute catastrophic spinal injuries are those associated with unstable fractures and dislocations, intervertebral disc herniation, and transient quadriplegia. These most commonly affect the cervical spine, but also affect the thoracolumbar spine (the thoracic and lumbar vertebrae) and physis, or cause cervical cord neuropraxia and sometimes spinal cord injury without radiographic abnormality (SCIWORA).

Response to a non-fatal catastrophic spinal cord injury by the patient varies by "social, economic, and educational background".

The most common initial response is depression. About 6% of patients with a spinal cord injury commit suicide, usually in the years immediately after sustaining the injury. By ten years after an injury, the rate of suicide is similar to that of the general population.

Many patients recover only partially from their injury, and must cope with paralysis or mental deficiency, usually requiring lifetime medical care.

About 90% of patients who are single when injured are still single five years after the injury. There is a high incidence of divorce and separation after an injury, though this decreases beyond the first year after injury.

Many catastrophic spinal cord injury patients improve their education. Immediately after injury, the average level of education is below that of the general population; fifteen years after injury, it is above that of the general population.

Survivors of catastrophic injury may also have catastrophic facial injuries, such as fractured facial bones, particularly those from events associated with ice hockey, cycling, and snowmobiling.

Medical Problems

Numerous secondary medical problems are associated with catastrophic spinal cord injury. These include cardiovascular complications, such as deep vein thrombosis, pulmonary embolism, orthostatic hypotension, bradycardia, autonomic dysreflexia, altered thermoregulation, and changes to cardiac function as a result of injury to the sympathetic nervous system.

Other problems may include pulmonary and gastrointestinal problems, heterotopic ossification, osteoporosis, and other pathologic fractures. Pneumonia is a common cause of death among patients with spinal cord injuries.

A skull fracture occurs when a bone in the skull breaks, and may penetrate the brain, tearing arteries, veins, or meninges, leading to the functional impairment of walking, communication, thinking, or feeling. Cerebral lacerations (tearing of brain tissue) or cerebral contusions (bruising of brain tissue) usually damage the cerebral cortex, resulting in permanent neurological deficits.

Life Care Plan

A life care plan is established for the patient to address the patient's needs. It is an individualized document describing the services, support, equipment, and ancillary requirements for the patient that is updated to reflect changes in the patient's condition. It usually contains target outcomes, dates, and timelines.

Components of the life care plan may include:

- architectural renovations to the patient's home, including tub, toilet, and ingress and egress
- transportation, such as an adaptive van
- assistive technology and adaptive equipment, including wheelchairs
- case management
- supervisory care and nursing
- medication, medical supplies (such as catheters), and medical equipment

- facility care and services
- home care and services

This is in addition to information regarding surgical intervention and treatment, diagnostic testing, therapeutic interventions (speech therapy, rehabilitation, etc.), counselling, and dealing with complications. It may also include educational and vocational services.

In the United States, 2.55% of hospitalized catastrophic injury patients enroll in Medicaid to cover their medical bills. In *Catastrophic Injuries in Sports and Recreation: Causes and Prevention : A Canadian Study*, Charles Tator states that the average case of non-fatal catastrophic injury costs about $7.5 million (Canadian dollars, normalized to 2006) in lost earnings, lifetime care, and rehabilitation services, and cost the economy of Ontario about $2.125 billion annually.

Prevention

One paradigm used in injury prevention is the Haddon Matrix developed by William Haddon Jr. of the National Highway Safety Bureau in the late 1960s. The matrix was designed to categorize highway safety phenomena, and applied a public health model to traffic-related epidemiology. It consists of ten strategies that are implemented based on temporality, that is pre-event strategies (primary prevention), event strategies (secondary prevention), and post-event strategies (tertiary prevention). The purpose of injury prevention is to decrease the "burden of injury to the individual and to society", which includes mortality, morbidity, disability, and economic cost.

The ten strategies are:

- pre-event strategies
  - prevent the creation of the hazard
  - reduce the amount of hazard
  - prevent the release of the hazard
  - modify the rate or distribution of release of the hazard
- event strategies
  - separate the potential victims from the hazard, in time or space
  - separate the potential victims from the hazard with a barrier
  - modify the hazard

  - improve individual resistance to the hazard
- post-event strategies
  - counter incurred damage
  - stabilize, treat, and rehabilitate the injured individual

In *Catastrophic Head Injuries in High School and Collegiate Sports*, Frederick Mueller states that the frequency of catastrophic injuries may be reduced by:

- requiring all participants to submit medical histories and have an obligatory pre-participation examination
- requiring all schools, colleges, and universities to have a certified athletic trainer on faculty
- enforcement of game rules by officials and coaches, and player education about head contact
- removing a player exhibiting symptoms of concussion or head trauma from a game
- educating players, parents, coaches about the symptoms of head injury and dangers of recurrent injury
- athletic trainer must be prepared to respond to a catastrophic injury event

Preparation for a catastrophic injury event includes a written emergency plan, which should incorporate an evacuation, transportation and communication plan, as well as notifying hospital emergency departments about game and practice schedules for teams and clubs. Response to a catastrophic injury event should reduce its severity, such as via the administration of first aid. In *Catastrophic Injuries in Sports and Recreation: Causes and Prevention : A Canadian Study*, Charles Tator states that effective injury prevention programs involve education, engineering, and rule enforcement. Education is intended to inform the participants of potential dangers of risky behaviour in the activity, and engineering "involved modifying the environment to create safer surroundings", such as maintaining playing fields or improving the design of equipment.

Response

Sports organizations, leagues, and associations have integrated a catastrophic injury plan as part of their emergency action and emergency management plans, and have also changed rules to prevent or reduce the incidence of catastrophic injuries. Such plans include a notification system, which may be used to contact the family of the injured athlete, athletic coordinators, officials, legal and risk management offices, and institutional insurance carriers.

It may also include the formation of a catastrophic injury team, which may include athletic directors, head athletic trainer, team physicians, legal counsel, and media relations.

In 1985, the National Collegiate Athletic Association created an insurance plan for member institutions to provide benefits for student athletes who sustain a catastrophic injury, in response to an increase in workers' compensation claims filed by students. This was designed to protect member institutions "against the sudden and substantial costs of injury benefits", typically obtained by the student via worker's compensation claims and litigation. The injured student receives benefits immediately and does not incur litigation costs, but retains the right to litigation in cases of negligence by the institution. In 2005, 25% of funds for insurance claim payouts were associated with cheerleading.

The National Federation of High School Associations instituted a medical plan for high school athletic associations and their member schools and districts. This allows a catastrophically injured student athlete to receive "medical, rehabilitation, and work-loss benefits" until death by waiving rights to litigation. The institution thereby need not invest the human and financial resources associated with litigation, in addition to a potential award to the plaintiff, and the student receives immediate and lifelong benefits.

Athletic associations, organizations, and leagues update their rules based on research regarding catastrophic injuries. The amount of enforcement of the rules may explain variations in incidence of catastrophic injuries between jurisdictions.

Litigation

In Canada, as of May 2012 the largest award to a plaintiff of a catastrophic brain injury was $18.4 million, and the largest award to a plaintiff of a catastrophic spinal cord injury was $12.33 million.

In South Africa, the largest malpractice settlement for the Medical Protection Society as of 2011 was for R17 million, awarded to a patient who suffered catastrophic neurological damage as a result of a surgical procedure.

Anterior Cruciate Ligament Injury

Anterior cruciate ligament injury occurs when the biomechanical limits of the ligament are exceeded (over-stretched). The anterior cruciate ligament (ACL) is an important internal stabilizer of the knee joint. The primary function of the ACL is to prevent hyperextension; its secondary function is to restrain tibial rotation and varus/valgus stress.

ACL injury is most commonly a non-contact injury involving a sudden stop or twisting movement, such as a dismount from a layup in basketball. ACL injury occurs more frequently in athletes than in the general population and is prevalent in alpine skiing, association football, American football, Australian rules football, basketball, rugby, professional wrestling, martial arts, and gymnastics. It is also known to be about three times more common in women than men.

The consequences of the injury depend on how much the stability of the knee is affected, and the extent to which other structures have been involved. If instability is evident, particularly rotatory instability, then the menisci may get injured; this may lead to progressive, degenerative, arthritis of the knee.

Signs and Symptoms

An individual may feel or hear a "pop" in their knee during a twisting movement or rapid deceleration, followed by an inability to continue participation in the sport and early swelling from hemarthrosis. This combination is said to indicate a 90% probability of rupture of the anterior cruciate ligament. An individual may experience instability in the knee once they resume walking and other activities, and they may feel their knee is "giving out".

Causes

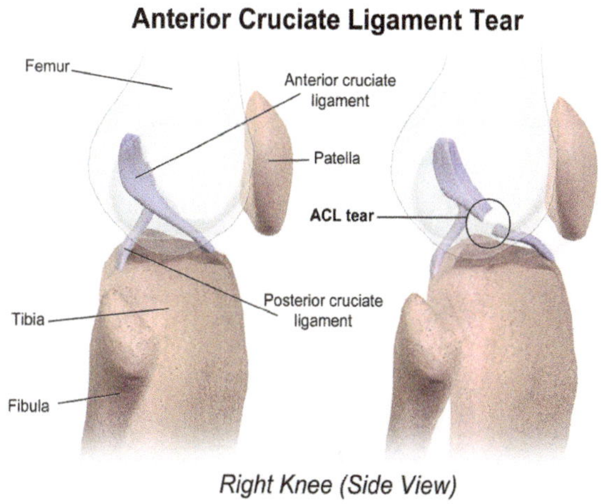

ACL Tear

ACL injury is most commonly a non-contact injury that occurs when an individual stops suddenly or plants his or her foot hard into the ground (*cutting*). ACL injury also has been linked to *heavy* or stiff-legged landing; the knee rotating while landing, especially when the knee is in an unnatural position.

Significantly, many ACL injuries occur in athletes landing flat on their heels. This movement directs the forces directly up the tibia into the knee, while the straight-knee position places the anterior femoral condyle on the back-slanted portion of the tibia. The resultant forward slide of the tibia relative to the femur is restrained primarily by the now-vulnerable ACL.

ACL injuries also can be caused by direct contact or trauma, such as in a motor vehicle collision or from a tackle in football. A severe form of ACL injury caused by direct contact is called the "unhappy triad," also known as the "terrible triad," or "O'Donaghue's triad." The "unhappy triad" involves injury of the anterior cruciate ligament, the medial collateral ligament, and the medial meniscus.

Risk Factors

Sex-related Differences

Women in sports such as association football, basketball, and tennis are significantly more prone to ACL injuries than men. The discrepancy has been attributed to gender differences in anatomy, general muscular strength, reaction time of muscle contraction and coordination, and training techniques.

Gender differences in ACL injury rates become evident when specific sports are compared. A review of NCAA data has found relative rates of injury per 1000 athlete exposures as follows:

- Men's basketball 0.07, women's basketball 0.23
- Men's lacrosse 0.12, women's lacrosse 0.17
- Men's football 0.09, women's football 0.28

The highest rate of ACL injury in women occurred in gymnastics, with a rate of injury per 1000 athlete exposures of 0.33 Of the four sports with the highest ACL injury rates, three were women's – gymnastics, basketball and soccer.

According to recent studies, female athletes are two to eight times more likely to strain their anterior cruciate ligament (ACL) in sports that involve cutting and jumping as compared to men who play the same particular sports (soccer, basketball, and volleyball). Differences between males and females identified as potential causes are the active muscular protection of the knee joint, the greater Q angle putting more medial torque on the knee joint, relative ligament laxity caused by differences in hormonal activity from estrogen and relaxin, intercondylar notch dimensions, and muscular strength.

Hormonal and Anatomic Differences

Before puberty, there is no observed difference in frequency of ACL tears between the sexes. Changes in sex hormone levels, specifically elevated levels of estrogen and relaxin in females during the menstrual cycle, have been hypothesized as causing predisposition of ACL ruptures. This is because they may increase joint laxity and extensibility of the soft tissues surrounding the knee joint. Additionally, female pelvises widen during puberty through the influence of sex hormones. This wider pelvis requires the femur to angle toward the knees. This angle towards the knee is referred to as the Q angle. The average Q angle for men is 14 degrees and the average for women is 17 degrees. Steps can be taken to reduce this Q angle, such as using orthotics. The relatively wider female hip and widened Q angle may lead to an increased likelihood of ACL tears in women.

ACL, Muscular Stiffness and Strength

During puberty, sex hormones also affect the remodeled shape of soft tissues throughout the body. The tissue remodeling results in female ACLs that are smaller and will fail (i.e. tear) at lower loading forces, and differences in ligament and muscular stiffness between men and women. Women's knees are less stiff than men's during muscle activation. Force applied to a less stiff knee is more likely to result in ACL tears.

In addition, the quadriceps femoris muscle is an antagonist to the ACL. According to a study done on female athletes at the University of Michigan, 31% of female athletes recruited the quadriceps femoris muscle first as compared to 17% in males. Because of the elevated contraction of the quadriceps femoris muscle during physical activity, an increased strain is placed onto the ACL due to the "tibial translation anteriorly".

Ligament Dominance

The increased risk of anterior cruciate ligament injury among female athletes is best predicted by the motion and loading of the knee during performance situations. The ligament dominance theory suggests that females typically perform athletic movements with greater knee valgus angles. A greater amount of stress is placed on the ACL in these situations because there is high activation of the quadriceps muscles despite limited knee flexion, limited hip flexion, greater hip adduction, and a large knee adductor moment. Additionally, females typically land with their tibia rotated internally or externally. As a result of increased knee valgus stress, ground reaction forces are greater and laterally directed.

Quadriceps Dominance

Ligament dominance is observed when there is excessive movement in the frontal plane to accommodate limited movement in the sagittal plane. This is caused by weakness in the hamstring muscles or reliance on the strength of the quadriceps muscles. This quadriceps dominance theory identifies when the hamstring muscles are notably weaker than the quadriceps muscles. As a result, knee stability in performance situations depends on the quadriceps due to a discrepancy in the pattern in recruiting quadriceps and hamstring muscles.

Trunk and Leg dominance

Other theories used to explain the increased risk of ACL injury among female athletes include the trunk dominance and leg dominance theories. Trunk dominance suggests that males typically exhibit greater control of the trunk in performance situations as evidenced by greater activation of the internal oblique muscle. Leg dominance suggests that females exhibit greater kinematic leg asymmetry in knee valgus angles, hip abduction, and ankle abduction in performance situations.

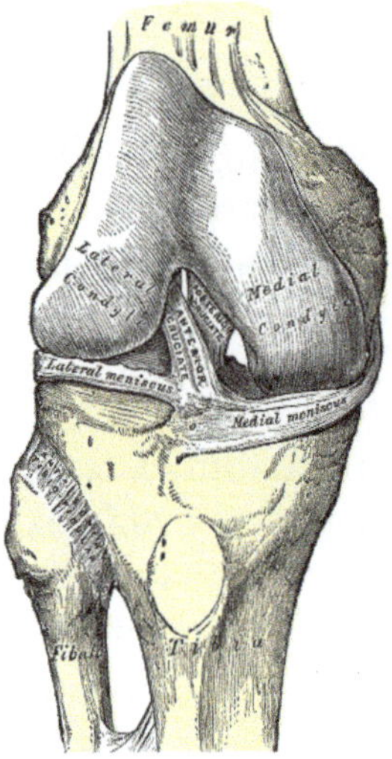

Right knee, front, showing interior ligaments

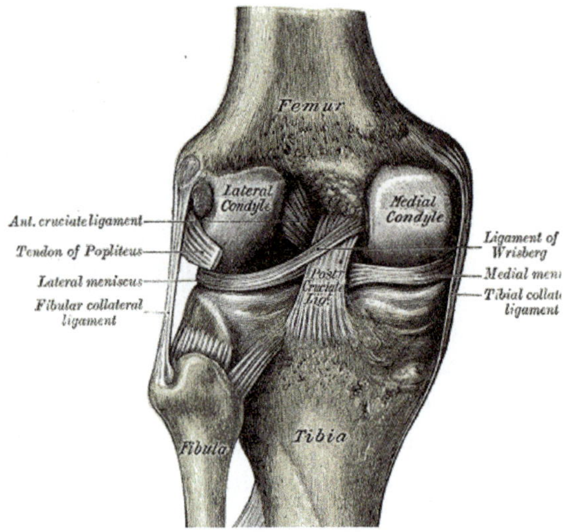

Left knee, behind, showing interior ligaments

Diagnosis

Manual Tests

The pivot-shift test, anterior drawer test, and Lachman test are used during the clinical examination of suspected ACL injury. The Lachman test is recognized by most authorities as the most reliable and sensitive test, and usually superior to the anterior drawer test.

An ACL tear can present with a popping sound heard after impact, swelling after a couple of hours, severe pain when bending the knee, and buckling or locking of the knee during movement.

Though clinical examination in experienced hands can be accurate, the diagnosis is usually confirmed by using an arthrometer or MRI, which have greatly lessened the need for diagnostic arthroscopy and which have a higher accuracy than clinical examination. It may also permit visualization of other structures which may have been coincidentally involved, such as a meniscus, or collateral ligament, or posterolateral corner of the knee joint.

Laximetry

Laximetry is a reliable technique for diagnosing a torn anterior cruciate ligament.

MRI Scan

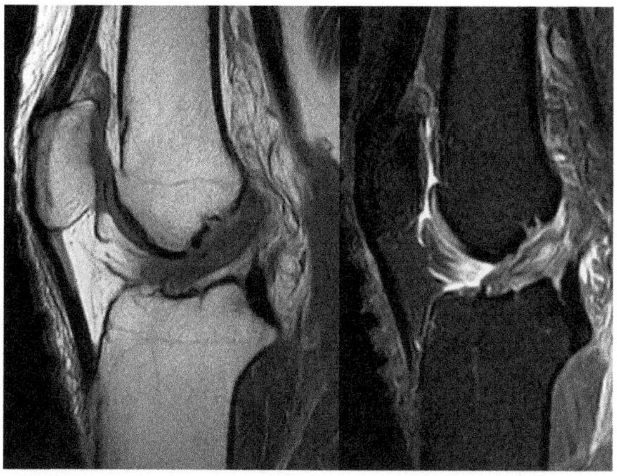

Anterior cruciate ligament tear seen on MRI. T1 left, right PDW

The MRI is perhaps the most used technique for diagnosing the state of the Anterior Cruciate Ligament but it not always the most reliable. In some cases the Anterior Cruciate Ligament can indeed not be seen because of the blood surrounding it.

Prevention

Interest in reducing non-contact ACL injury has been intense and the observed, increased, liability of the female gender in some sports has added to this. The International Olympic Committee, after a comprehensive review of preventive strategies, has stated that injury prevention programs have an effect on reducing injuries that is measurable, and that applies particularly to women. Further, paying attention to the balance of strength between hamstrings and quadriceps will help prevent the anterior cruciate ligament from being overpowered by over-emphasized quadriceps strength. It is also stressed that landing forces should be reduced together with emphasizing proper landing technique. It has been previously reported that landing on the heel, rather than forefoot with progressive transfer of weight to the heel, is potentially injurious to the ACL because of the hyperextension forces created. The closer the knee is to full extension, the more likely this is to occur.

Accordingly, it is generally recommended that injury prevention programs stress these principles.

Treatment

The term for non-surgical treatment for ACL rupture is "conservative management", and it often includes physical therapy and using a knee brace. Instability associated with ACL deficiency increases the risk of other knee injuries such as a torn meniscus, so sports with cutting and twisting motions are problematic and surgery is often recommended in those circumstances.

Patients who have suffered an ACL injury should be evaluated for other injuries that often occur in combination with an ACL tear and include cartilage/meniscus injuries, bone bruises, PCL tears, posterolateral injuries and collateral ligament injuries.

Conservative

A torn ACL is less likely to restrict the movement of the knee. When tears to the ACL are not repaired it can sometimes cause damage to the cartilage inside the knee because with the torn ACL the tibia and femur bone are more likely to rub against each other. Immediately after the tear of the ACL, the person should rest the knee, ice it every 15 to 20 minutes, provide compression on the knee, and then elevate above the heart; this process helps decrease the swelling and reduce the pain. The form of treatment is determined based on the severity of the tear on the ligament. Small tears in the ACL may just require several months of rehab in order to strengthen the surrounding muscles, the hamstring and the quadriceps, so that these muscles can compensate for the torn ligament. Falls associated with knee instability may require the use of a specific brace to stabilize the knee. Women are more likely to experience falls associated with the knee giving way. Sudden falls can be associated with further complications such as fractures and head injury.

Surgery

If surgery is decided upon, either because obvious instability interferes with activities of daily living, or because the knee is subject to repeated, severe, provocative maneuvers, such as the case of the competitive athlete involved in cutting and rapid deceleration etc., then several issues need to be decided upon.

- Timing. Immediate repair is usually avoided and initial swelling and inflammatory reaction allowed to subside.
- Choice of graft material, autograft or allograft.
- Choice of anterior cruciate ligament augmentation, patellar tendon or hamstring tendon.

These issues are fully explored in ACL Reconstruction.

Epidemiology

There are around 200,000 ACL tears each year in the United States, with over 100,000 ACL reconstruction surgeries per year. Over 95% of ACL reconstructions are performed in the outpatient setting. The most common procedures performed during ACL reconstruction are partial meniscectomy and chondroplasty.

Young Athletes

High school athletes are at increased risk for ACL tears when compared to non-athletes. This risk increases with certain types of sports. Among high school girls, the sport with the highest risk of ACL tear is soccer, followed by basketball and lacrosse. The highest risk sport for boys was basketball, followed by lacrosse and soccer. Children and young athletes may benefit from early surgical reconstruction after ACL injury. Young athletes who have early surgical reconstruction of their torn ACL are more likely to return to their previous level of athletic ability when compared to those who underwent delayed surgery or nonoperative treatment. They are also less likely to experience instability in their knee if the undergo early surgery.

Shin Splints

Shin splints, also known as medial tibial stress syndrome (MTSS), is defined by the American Academy of Orthopaedic Surgeons as "pain along the inner edge of the shinbone (tibia)." Shin splints are usually caused by repeated trauma to the connective muscle tissue surrounding the tibia. They are a common injury affecting athletes who engage in running sports or other forms of physical activity, including running and jumping. They are characterized by general pain in the lower region of the leg between the knee and the ankle. Shin splints injuries are specifically located in the middle to lower thirds of the anterior or lateral part of the tibia, which is the larger of two bones comprising the lower leg.

Shin splints are the most prevalent lower leg injury and affect a broad range of individuals. It affects mostly runners and accounts for approximately 13% to 17% of all running-related injuries. High school age runners see shin splints injury rates of approximately 13%. Aerobic dancers have also been known to suffer from shin splints, with injury rates as high as 22%. Military personnel undergoing basic training experience shin splints injury rates between 4-8%.

Causes

While the exact cause is unknown, shin splints can be attributed to the overloading of the lower leg due to biomechanical irregularities resulting in an increase in stress exerted on the tibia. A sudden increase in intensity or frequency in activity level fatigues muscles too quickly to properly help absorb shock, forcing the tibia to absorb most of that shock. This stress is associated with the onset of shin splints. Muscle imbalance, including weak core muscles, inflexibility and tightness of lower leg muscles, including the gastrocnemius, soleus, and plantar muscles (commonly the flexor digitorum longus) can increase the possibility of shin splints. The pain associated with shin splints is caused from a disruption of Sharpey's fibres that connect the medial soleus fascia through the periosteum of the tibia where it inserts into the bone. With repetitive stress, the impact forces eccentrically fatigue the soleus and create repeated tibial bending or bowing, contributing to shin splints. The impact is made worse by running uphill, downhill, on uneven terrain, or on hard surfaces. Improper footwear, including worn-out shoes, can also contribute to shin splints.

Diagnosis

Shin splints can be diagnosed by a physician after taking a thorough history and performing a complete physical examination. The physical examination uses gentle pressure to determine whether there is tenderness over a 4–6 inch section on the lower, inside shin area. The pain has been described as a dull ache to an intense pain that increases during exercise, and some individuals experience swelling in the pain area. People who have previously had shin splints are more likely to have it again.

Vascular and neurological examinations produce normal results in patients with shin splints. Radiographies and three-phase bone scans are recommended to differentiate between shin splints and other causes of chronic leg pain. Bone scintigraphy and MRI scans can be used to differentiate between stress fractures and shin splints.

It is important to differentiate between different lower leg pain injuries, including shin splints, stress fractures, compartment syndrome, nerve entrapment, and popliteal artery entrapment syndrome. These conditions often have many overlapping symptoms which makes a final diagnosis difficult, and correct diagnosis is needed to determine the most appropriate treatment.

If shin splints are not treated properly, or if exercise is resumed too early or aggressively, shin splints can become permanent.

Treatment

Typical treatments include rest, ice, strengthening and gradually returning to activity. Rest and ice work to allow the tibia to recover from sudden, high levels of stress and reduce inflammation and pain levels. It is important to significantly reduce any pain or swelling before returning to activity. Strengthening exercises should be performed after pain has subsided, on lower leg and hip muscles. Individuals should gradually return to activity, beginning with a short and low intensity level. Over multiple weeks, they can slowly work up to normal activity level. It is important to decrease activity level if any pain returns. Individuals should consider running on other surfaces besides asphalt, such as grass, to decrease the amount of force the lower leg must absorb. Orthoses and insoles help to offset biomechanical irregularities, like pronation, and help to support the arch of the foot. Other conservative interventions include footwear refitting, orthotics, manual therapy, balance training (e.g. using a balance board), cortisone injections, and calcium and vitamin D supplementation.

Less common forms of treatment for more severe cases of shin splints include extracorporeal shockwave therapy (ESWT) and surgery. Surgery is only performed in extreme cases where more conservative options have been tried for at least a year. However, surgery does not guarantee 100% recovery.

Epidemiology

Risk factors for developing shin splints include:

- Excessive pronation at subtalar joint
- Excessively tight calf muscles (which can cause excessive pronation)
- Engaging the medial shin muscle in excessive amounts of eccentric muscle activity
- Undertaking high-impact exercises on hard, noncompliant surfaces (ex: running on asphalt or concrete)
- Smoking and low fitness level

While medial tibial stress syndrome is the most common form of shin splints, compartment syndrome and stress fractures are also common forms of shin splints. Females are 1.5 to 3.5 times more likely to progress to stress fractures from shin splints. This is due in part to females having a higher incidence of diminished bone density and osteoporosis.

Boxer's Fracture

Boxer's Fracture is a colloquial term for a fracture of one of the metacarpal bones of the hand. Classically, the fracture occurs transversely across the neck of the bone, after the patient strikes an object with a closed fist. Alternate terms include scrapper's fracture or bar room fracture.

As these are colloquial terms, texts and medical dictionaries do not universally agree on precise meanings. Various authorities state that a "Boxer's fracture" means a break in specifically the second metacarpal bone or third metacarpal bone, with "Bar Room fracture" being specific to the fourth metacarpal bone or fifth metacarpal bone. Though some writers assert that Boxer's fracture and Bar Room fracture are distinct terms representing injuries to different bones, this distinction seems to have been lost over time and most medical professionals now describe any metacarpal fracture as a "Boxer's Fracture".

Signs and Symptoms

The symptoms are pain and tenderness in the specific location of the hand, which corresponds to the metacarpal bone around the knuckle. When a fracture occurs, there may be a snapping or popping sensation. There will be swelling of the hand along with discoloration or bruising in the affected area. Abrasions or lacerations of the hand are also likely to occur. The respective finger may be misaligned, and movement of that finger may be limited and painful.

Causes

Metacarpal fractures are usually caused by the impact of a clenched fist with a hard, immovable object, such as a skull or a wall. When a punch impacts with improper form, the force occurs at an angle towards the palm, creating a dorsal bend in the bone, ultimately causing the fracture when the bone is bent too far.

When a boxer punches with proper form, the knuckles of the second and third metacarpal align linearly with the articulating radius, followed linearly by the humerus. Due to the linear articulation of bones, the force is able to travel freely across these joints and bones and be dissipated without injury. Therefore, fractures of the second or third metacarpals are rare, with fractures of the 4th and 5th metacarpals comprising the vast majority of metacarpal fractures.

Diagnosis

Diagnosis by a doctor's examination is the most common, often confirmed by x-rays. X-ray is used to display the fracture and the angulations of the fracture. A CT scan may be done in very rare cases to provide a more detailed picture.

Prevention

Boxers and other combat athletes routinely use hand wraps and boxing gloves to help stabilize the hand, greatly reducing pain and risk of injury during impact. Proper punching form is the most important factor to prevent this type of fracture.

Treatment

Once injured, the subject will feel both the swelling and associated pain in the hand. Ice is applied to relieve pain and swelling. Any open wounds are cleansed to avoid infection. The injured hand must remain immobilized, to avoid moving the broken end of the bone, which can cause damage to the muscles, blood vessels, tendons, ligaments and nerves.

Conservative treatment is to apply a splint to immobilize the affected part of the hand and allow healing. If the broken parts of the bone are misaligned by more than 70 degrees, or if the physician is unable to reduce (realign) the fragments by manipulation, surgery may be required to place pins or plates in the bone to hold the pieces in place.

Prognosis for these fractures is generally good, with total healing time not exceeding 12 weeks. The first two weeks will show significantly reduced overall swelling, with improvement in clenching ability showing up first. Ability to extend the fingers in all directions appears to improve more slowly. Hard casts are rarely required, and soft casts or splints can be removed for brief periods of time to allow for cleaning and drying the skin underneath the splint. Pain from injury varies person to person as with most injuries cannot in all honesty be generalized. Depending on the individual a course of over the counter or narcotic pain medication will suffice. Muscle atrophy of 5 to 15 percent may be expected, with a rehabilitation period of approximately 4 months given adequate therapy. In the mildest of cases, full rehabilitation status can be achieved within 3 to 4 months.

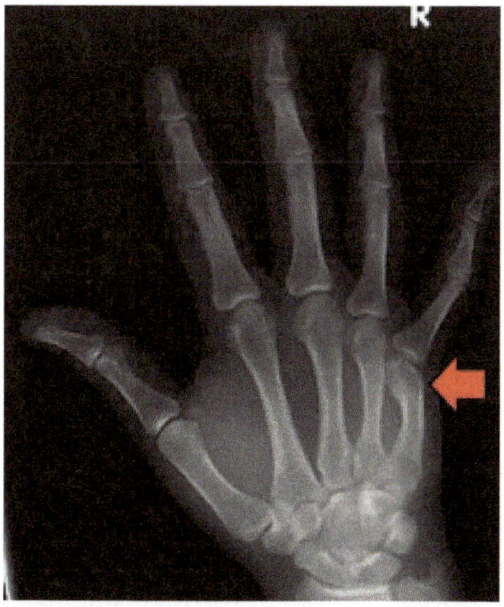

A healed fracture of the base of the 5th metacarpal

Epidemiology

Hand and wrist injuries are reported to account for fifteen to twenty percent of emergency room injuries, and metacarpal fractures represent a significant number of those injuries. Hand injuries of this sort are most prevalent among fifteen- to thirty-five-year-old males, and the fifth metacarpal is the one most commonly affected.

Males are nearly fifty percent more likely to sustain fracture from a punch mechanism than females. Male intentional punch injuries are correlated predominantly with social deprivation, while female punch intentional injuries show more correlation with psychiatric disorders.

Approximately 3.7 male hand injuries, per 1000, per year, and 1.3 female hand injuries, per 1000, per year, have been reported. Common mechanisms of injury are gender specific. Although the fiscal cost is not available, it can be asserted that the cost is reasonably significant per individual, depending on the cost of emergency care, immobilization, surgery, follow up doctors' visits, etc. in addition to the fiscal impact from loss of and/or limited work abilities.

Tennis Elbow

Tennis elbow or lateral epicondylitis is a condition in which the outer part of the elbow becomes sore and tender at the lateral epicondyle. The forearm muscles and tendons become damaged from repetitive overuse. This leads to pain and tenderness on the outside of the elbow.

Any activity, including playing tennis, that involves repetitive use of the extensor muscles of the forearm can cause acute or chronic tendonitis of the tendinous insertion of these muscles at the lateral epicondyle of the elbow. The condition is common in carpenters and laborers who swing a hammer or other tool with the forearm, and is similar to golfer's elbow, which affects the medial epicondyle on the inside of the elbow. Continuing activity after onset of the condition and avoiding mandatory rest may lead to permanent onset of pain and only treatable via surgery. German physician F. Runge is usually credited for the first description of the condition, calling it "writer's cramp" (*Schreibekrampf*) in 1873. Later, it was called "washer women's elbow". British surgeon Henry Morris published an article in *The Lancet* describing "lawn tennis arm" in 1883. The popular term "tennis elbow" first appeared the same year in a paper by H. P. Major, described as "lawn-tennis elbow".

Signs and Symptoms

- Pain on the outer part of the elbow (lateral epicondyle)
- Point tenderness over the lateral epicondyle—a prominent part of the bone on the outside of the elbow
- Pain from gripping and movements of the wrist, especially wrist extension and lifting movements
- Pain from activities that use the muscles that extend the wrist (e.g. pouring a container of liquid, lifting with the palm down, sweeping, especially where wrist movement is required)

Symptoms associated with tennis elbow include, but are not limited to: radiating pain from the outside of the elbow to the forearm and wrist, pain during extension of wrist, weakness of the forearm, a painful grip while shaking hands or torquing a doorknob, and not being able to hold relatively heavy items in the hand. The pain is similar to the condition known as *golfer's elbow*, but the latter occurs at the medial side of the elbow.

Causes

Tennis elbow is a type of repetitive strain injury resulting from tendon overuse and failed healing of the tendon. In addition, the extensor carpi radialis brevis muscle plays a key role.

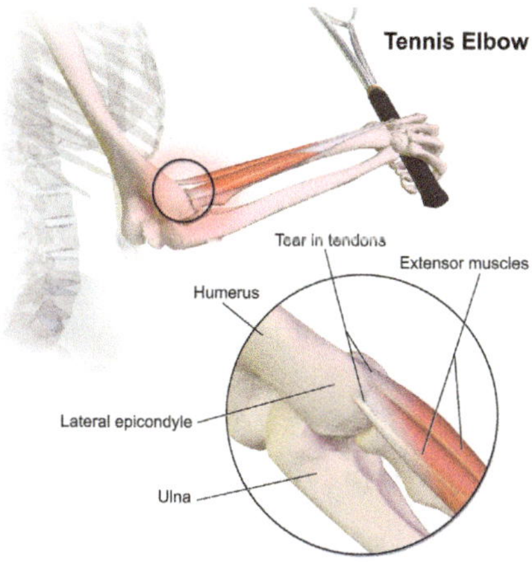

Location of tennis elbow

Early experiments suggested that tennis elbow was primarily caused by overexertion. However, studies show that trauma such as direct blows to the epicondyle, a sudden forceful pull, or forceful extension cause more than half of these injuries. Repeatedly mis-hitting a tennis ball in the early stages of learning the sport causes shock to the elbow joint and may contribute to contracting the condition.

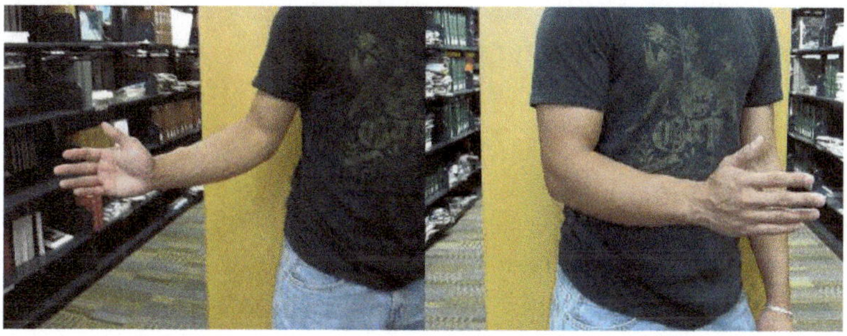

Example of repetitive movement that may cause tennis elbow

Cyriax proposes one explanation of how tennis elbow may come about. The hypothesis states that there are microscopic and macroscopic tears between the common extensor tendon and the periosteum of the lateral humeral epicondyle. An operation conducted in this study showed that 28 out of 39 patients showed tearing at the tendon cuff. Kaplan stated that the radial nerve was significantly involved in tennis elbow. He noted the constriction of the radial nerve by adhesions to the capsule of the radiohumeral joint and the short extensor muscle of the wrist. He found evidence that many differed in how they contracted tennis elbow. Disorders such as calcification of the rotator cuff, bicipital tendinitis, or carpal tunnel syndrome may increase chances of tennis elbow.

Pathophysiology

Histological findings include granulation tissue, microrupture, degenerative changes, and there is no traditional inflammation. As a consequence, "lateral elbow tendinopathy or tendinosis" is used instead of "lateral epicondylitis".

Examination of tennis elbow tissue reveals noninflammatory tissue, and therefore, the term "angio-fibroblastic tendinosis" is used.

Longitudinal sonogram of the lateral elbow displays thickening and heterogeneity of the common extensor tendon that is consistent with tendinosis, as the ultrasound reveals calcifications, intrasubstance tears, and marked irregularity of the lateral epicondyle. Although the term "epicondylitis" is frequently used to describe this disorder, most histopathologic findings of studies have displayed no evidence of an acute, or a chronic inflammatory process. Histologic studies have demonstrated that this condition is the result of tendon degeneration, which replaces normal tissue with a disorganized arrangement of collagen. Therefore, the disorder is more appropriately referred to as *tendinosis* or *tendinopathy* rather than *tendinitis*.

Colour Doppler ultrasound reveals structural tendon changes, with vascularity and hypo-echoic areas that correspond to the areas of pain in the extensor origin.

The pathophysiology of lateral epicondylitis is degenerative. Non-inflammatory, chronic degenerative changes of the origin of the extensor carpi radialis brevis (ECRB) muscle are identified in surgical pathology specimens. It is unclear if the pathology is affected by prior injection of corticosteroid.

Tennis players generally believe tennis elbow is caused by the repetitive nature of hitting thousands of tennis balls, which leads to tiny tears in the forearm tendon attachment at the elbow.

The extensor digiti minimi also has a small origin site medial to the elbow that this condition can affect. The muscle involves the extension of the little finger and some extension of the wrist allowing for adaption to "snap" or flick the wrist—usually associated with a racquet swing. Most often, the extensor muscles become painful due to tendon breakdown from over-extension. Improper form or movement allows for power in a swing to rotate through and around the wrist—creating a moment on that joint instead of the elbow joint or rotator cuff. This moment causes pressure to build impact forces to act on the tendon causing irritation and inflammation.

Some suggest an overuse theory advancing that the extensor carpi radialis brevis has a small origin and does transmit large forces through its tendon during repetitive grasping. It has also been implicated as being vulnerable during shear stress during all movements of the forearm.

At least one author questions that lateral epicondylitis is caused by repetitive microtrauma/overuse, maintaining the theory is likely overstated and lacks scientific support.

Other speculative risk factors for lateral epicondylitis include taking up tennis later in life, unaccustomed strenuous activity, decreased mental chronometry and speed and repetitive eccentric contraction of muscle (controlled lengthening of a muscle group).

Prevention

Another factor of tennis elbow injury is experience and ability. The proportion of players who reported a history of tennis elbow had an increased number of playing years. As for ability, poor technique increases the chance for injury much like any sport. Therefore, an individual must learn proper technique for all aspects of their sport. The competitive level of the athlete also affects the incidence of tennis elbow. Class A and B players had a significantly higher rate of tennis elbow occurrence compared to class C and novice players. However, an opposite, but not statistically significant, trend is observed for the recurrence of previous cases, with an increasingly higher rate as ability level decreases.

Other ways to prevent tennis elbow:

- Decrease the amount of playing time if already injured or feeling pain in outside part of the elbow.
- Stay in overall good physical shape.
- Strengthen the muscles of the forearm: (pronator quadratus, pronator teres, and supinator muscle)—the upper arm: (biceps, triceps)—and the shoulder (deltoid muscle) and upper back (trapezius). Increased muscular strength increases stability of joints such as the elbow.
- Like other sports, use equipment appropriate to your ability, body size, and muscular strength.
- Avoid any repetitive lifting or pulling of heavy objects (especially over your head)

Vibration dampeners (otherwise known as "gummies") are not believed to be a reliable preventative measure. Rather, proper weight distribution in the racket is thought to be a more viable option in negating shock.

Diagnosis

To diagnose tennis elbow, the physician performs a battery of tests in which he places pressure on the affected area while asking the patient to move the elbow, wrist, and fingers. X-rays can confirm and distinguish possibilities of existing causes of pain that are unrelated to tennis elbow, such as fracture or arthritis. Medical ultrasonography and magnetic resonance imaging (MRI) are other valuable tools for diagnosis but are frequently avoided due to the high cost. MRI screening can confirm excess fluid and swelling in the affected region in the elbow, such as the connecting point between the forearm bone and the extensor carpi radialis brevis.

Diagnosis is made by clinical signs and symptoms that are discrete and characteristic. With the elbow fully extended, the patient feels points of tenderness over the affected point on the elbow—which is the origin of the extensor carpi radialis brevis muscle from the lateral epicondyle (extensor carpi radialis brevis origin). There is also pain with passive wrist flexion and resistive wrist extension (Cozen's test). Resisted middle finger extension might indicate the involvement of Extensor Digitorum also. These tests shall be used to measure the prognosis of the condition.

Depending upon severity and quantity of multiple tendon injuries that have built up, the extensor carpi radialis brevis may not be fully healed by conservative treatment. Nirschl defines four stages of lateral epicondylitis, showing the introduction of permanent damage beginning at Stage 2.

1. Inflammatory changes that are reversible
2. Nonreversible pathologic changes to origin of the extensor carpi radialis brevis muscle
3. Rupture of ECRB muscle origin
4. Secondary changes such as fibrosis or calcification.

Treatment

Evidence for the treatment of lateral epicondylitis before 2010 was poor. There were clinical trials addressing many proposed treatments, but the trials were of poor quality.

A 2009 study looked at using eccentric exercise with a rubber bar in addition to standard treatment: the trial was stopped after 8 weeks because the improvement using the bar for therapy was so significant. Based on small sample size and a follow-up only 7 weeks from commencement of treatment, the study shows short-term improvements. This along with other studies allowed doctors to conclude that approximately 80-95% of all tennis elbow cases can be treated without surgery. However, long-term results have not yet been determined.

In some cases, severity of tennis elbow symptoms mend without any treatment, within six to 24 months. Tennis elbow left untreated can lead to chronic pain that degrades quality of daily living.

Physical

There are several recommendations regarding prevention, treatment, and avoidance of recurrence that are largely speculative including stretches and progressive strengthening exercises to prevent re-irritation of the tendon and other exercise measures.

One way to help treat minor cases of tennis elbow is to simply relax the affected arm.

The rest lets stress and tightness within the forearm slowly relax and eventually have the arm in working condition—in a day or two, depending on the case.

Evidence from the Tyler study suggests that eccentric exercise using a rubber bar is highly effective at eliminating pain and increasing strength. The exercise involves grasping a rubber bar, twisting it, then slowly untwisting it.

Moderate evidence exists demonstrating that joint manipulation directed at the elbow and wrist and spinal manipulation directed at the cervical and thoracic spinal regions results in clinical changes to pain and function. There is also moderate evidence for short-term and mid-term effectiveness of cervical and thoracic spine manipulation as an add-on therapy to concentric and eccentric stretching plus mobilisation of wrist and forearm. Although not yet conclusive, the short-term analgesic effect of manipulation techniques may allow more vigorous stretching and strengthening exercises, resulting in a better and faster recovery process of the affected tendon in lateral epicondylitis.

Low level laser therapy, administered at specific doses and wavelengths directly to the lateral elbow tendon insertions, offers short-term pain relief and less disability in tennis elbow, both alone and in conjunction with an exercise regimen. Recently, dry needling has gained popularity to treat various types of tendinopathies and pain of muscular origin. Even in lateral epicondylitis, dry needling is widely used by physical therapists across the world. Proponents believe that dry needling causes a tiny local injury that brings about various desirable growth factors in the vicinity. Dry needling also aims at eliciting local twitch response (LTR) in the extensor muscles—as in some cases of tennis elbow the extensor muscles of the forearm would harbor trigger points, which itself could be a major source of pain.

Orthotic Devices

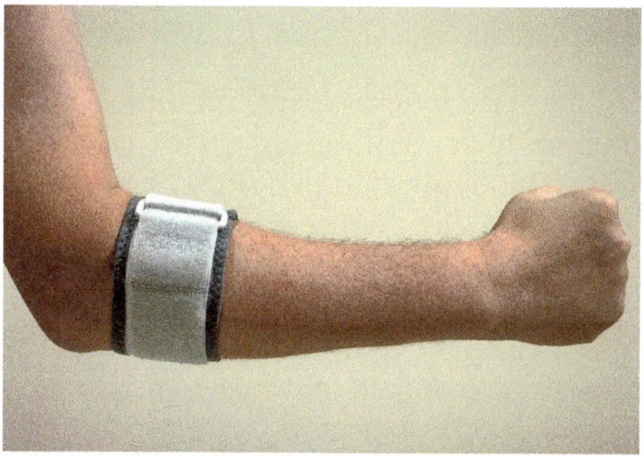

Counterforce orthosis reduces the elongation within the musculotendinious fibers

Orthosis is a device externally used on the limb to improve the function or reduce the pain. Orthotics are useful therapeutic interventions for initial therapy of tennis elbow.

There are two main types of orthoses prescribed for this problem: counterforce elbow orthoses and wrist extension orthoses.

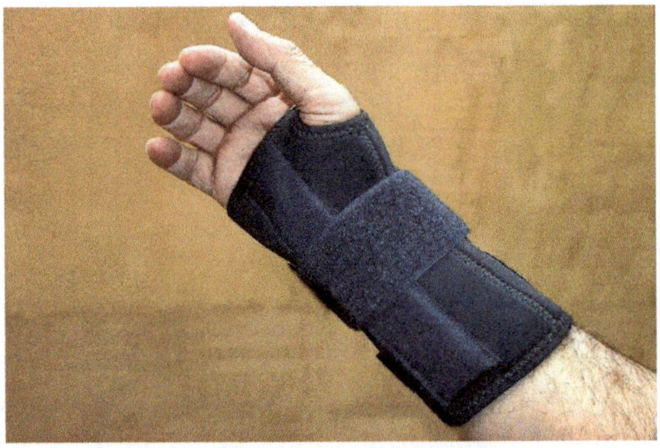

Wrist extensor orthosis reduces the overloading strain at the lesion area

Counterforce orthosis has a circumferential structure surrounding the arm. This orthosis usually has a strap which applies a binding force over the origin of the wrist extensors. The applied force by orthosis reduces the elongation within the musculotendinious fibers. Wrist extensor orthosis maintains the wrist in the slight extension. This position reduces the overloading strain at the lesion area.

Studies indicated both type of orthoses improve the hand function and reduce the pain in people with tennis elbow.

Medication

Although anti-inflammatories are a commonly prescribed treatment for tennis elbow, the evidence for their effect is usually anecdotal with only limited studies showing a benefit. A systematic review found that topical non-steroidal anti-inflammatory drugs (NSAIDs) may improve pain in the short term (up to 4 weeks) but was unable to draw firm conclusions due to methodological issues. Evidence for oral NSAIDs is mixed.

Evidence is poor for long term improvement from injections of any type, whether corticosteroids, botulinum toxin, prolotherapy or other substances. Corticosteroid injection may be effective in the short term however are of little benefit after a year, compared to a wait and see approach. A recent randomized control trial comparing the effect of corticosteroid injection, physiotherapy, or a combination of corticosteroid injection and physiotherapy found that patients treated with corticosteroid injection versus placebo had lower complete recovery or improvement at 1 year (Relative risk 0.86). Patients that received corticosteroid injection also had a higher recurrence rate at 1 year versus placebo (54% versus 12%, relative risk 0.23). Complications from repeated steroid injections include skin problems such as hypopigmentation and fat atrophy leading to indentation of the skin around the injection site. Botulinum toxin type A to paralyze the forearm extensor muscles in those with chronic tennis elbow that has not improved with conservative measures may be viable.

Surgery

In recalcitrant cases surgery may be an option. Surgical methods include:

- Lengthening, release, debridement, or repair of the origin of the extrinsic extensor muscles of the hand at the lateral epicondyle
- Rotation of the anconeus muscle
- Denervation of the lateral epicondyle
- Decompression of the posterior interosseous nerve

Surgical techniques for lateral epicondylitis can be done by open surgery, percutaneous surgery or arthroscopic surgery, with no evidence that any particular type is better or worse than another.

Prognosis

Response to initial therapy is common, but so is relapse (25% to 50%) and/or prolonged, moderate discomfort (40%).

Epidemiology

In tennis players, about 39.7% have reported current or previous problems with their elbow. Less than one quarter (24%) of these athletes under the age of 50 reported that the tennis elbow symptoms were "severe" and "disabling," while 42% were over the age of 50. More women (36%) than men (24%) considered their symptoms severe and disabling. Tennis elbow is more prevalent in individuals over 40, where there is about a four-fold increase among men and two-fold increase among women. Tennis elbow equally affects both sexes and, although men have a marginally higher overall prevalence rate as compared to women, this is not consistent within each age group, nor is it a statistically significant difference.

Playing time is a significant factor in tennis elbow occurrence, with increased incidence with increased playing time being greatery for respondents under 40. Individuals over 40 who played over two hours doubled their chance of injury. Those under 40 increased it 3.5 fold compared to those who played less than two hours per day.

Golfer's Elbow

Golfer's elbow, or medial epicondylitis, is tendinosis of the medial epicondyle on the inside of the elbow. It is in some ways similar to tennis elbow, which affects the outside at the lateral epicondyle.

The anterior forearm contains several muscles that are involved with flexing the digits of the hand, and flexing and pronating the wrist. The tendons of these muscles come together in a common tendinous sheath, which originates from the medial epicondyle of the humerus at the elbow joint. In response to minor injury, or sometimes for no obvious reason at all, this point of insertion becomes inflamed.

Causes

The condition is called *Golfer's Elbow* because in making a golf swing this tendon is stressed, especially if a non-overlapping (baseball style) grip is used; many people, however, who develop the condition have never handled a golf club. It is also sometimes called *Pitcher's Elbow* due to the same tendon being stressed by the throwing of objects such as a baseball, but this usage is much less frequent. Other names are *Climber's Elbow* and *Little League Elbow*: all of the flexors of the fingers and the pronators of the forearm insert at the medial epicondyle of the humerus to include: pronator teres, flexor carpi radialis, flexor carpi ulnaris, flexor digitorum superficialis, and palmaris longus; making this the most common elbow injury for rock climbers, whose sport is very grip intensive. The pain is normally caused due to stress on the tendon as a result of the large amount of grip exerted by the digits and torsion of the wrist which is caused by the use and action of the cluster of muscles on the condyle of the ulna.

Epicondylitis is much more common on the lateral side of the elbow (tennis elbow), rather than the medial side. In most cases, its onset is gradual and symptoms often persist for weeks before patients seek care. In golfer's elbow, pain at the medial epicondyle is aggravated by resisted wrist flexion and pronation, which is used to aid diagnosis. On the other hand, tennis elbow is indicated by the presence of lateral epicondylar pain precipitated by resisted wrist extension. Although the condition is poorly understood at a cellular and molecular level, there are hypotheses that point to apoptosis and autophagic cell death as causes of chronic lateral epicondylitis. The cell death may decrease the muscle density and cause a snowball effect in muscle weakness - this susceptibility can compromise a muscle's ability to maintain its integrity. So athletes, like pitchers, must work on preventing this cell death via flexibility training and other preventive measures.

Treatment

Non-specific treatments include:

- Non-steroidal anti-inflammatory drugs (NSAIDs): ibuprofen, naproxen or aspirin
- Heat or ice
- A counter-force brace or "elbow strap" to reduce strain at the elbow epicondyle, to limit pain provocation and to protect against further damage.

Before anesthetics and steroids are used, conservative treatment with an occupational therapist may be attempted. Before therapy can commence, treatment such as the common rest, ice, compression and elevation (R.I.C.E.) will typically be used. This will help to decrease the pain and inflammation; rest will alleviate discomfort because golfer's elbow is an overuse injury. The patient can use a tennis elbow splint for compression. A pad can be placed anteromedially on the proximal forearm. The splint is made in 30–45 degrees of elbow flexion. A daytime elbow pad also may be useful, by limiting additional trauma to the nerve.

Therapy will include a variety of exercises for muscle/tendon reconditioning, starting with stretching and gradual strengthening of the flexor-pronator muscles. Strengthening will slowly begin with isometrics and progresses to eccentric exercises helping to extend the range of motion back to where it once was. After the strengthening exercises, it is common for the patient to ice the area.

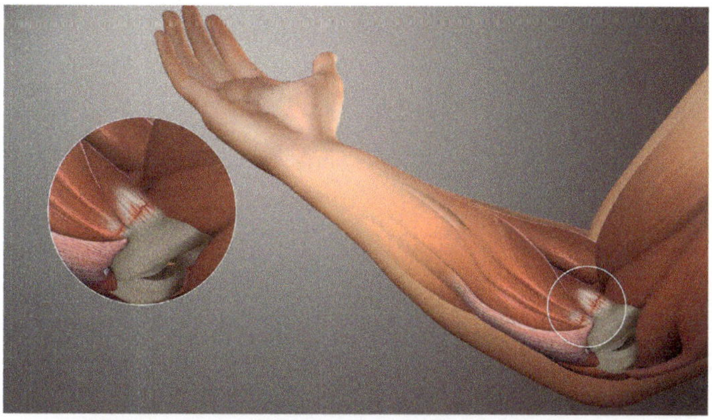

Still shot from a 3D medical animation illustrating
Golfer's elbow affecting the medial epicondyle on the lower inside of the joint

Simple analgesic medication has a place, as does more specific treatment with oral anti-inflammatory medications (NSAIDs). These will help control pain and any inflammation. A more invasive treatment is the injection into and around the inflamed and tender area of a long-acting glucocorticoid (steroid) agent. After causing an initial exacerbation of symptoms lasting 24 to 48 hours, this may produce an improvement of the condition in some five to seven days.

The ulnar nerve runs in the groove between the medial humeral epicondyle and the olecranon process of the ulna. It is most important that this nerve should not be damaged accidentally in the process of injecting a golfer's elbow.

If all else fails, epicondylar debridement (a surgery) may be effective. The ulnar nerve may also be decompressed surgically.

If the appropriate remediation steps are taken - rest, ice, and rehabilitative exercise and stretching - recovery may follow. Few patients will need to progress to steroid injection, and less than 10% will require surgical intervention.

Injuries in Netball

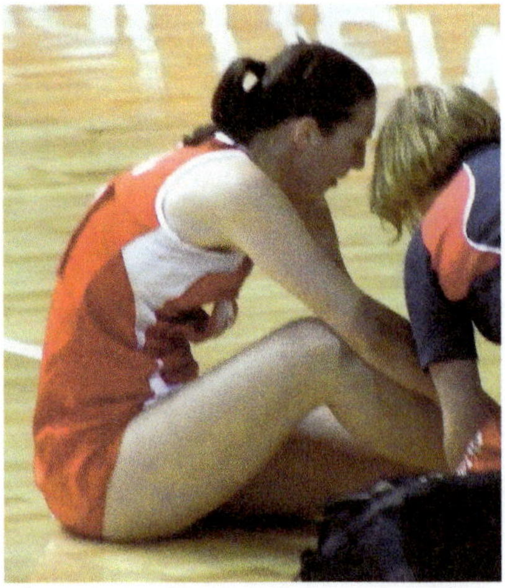

Rachel Dunn from Australia v England - Netball Test - Adelaide, October 2008 with an ankle injury

Netball is a sport that has one of the largest female participation rates within the commonwealth, most popular in the United Kingdom, Australia and New Zealand, with more than 20 million athletes participating in the sport. Netball is a ball sport played by two teams of seven players in which goals are scored by shooting the ball through a netted ring. Netball relies heavily on muscular endurance and bursts of rapid acceleration to "break free" from an opponent as well as, sudden and rapid change of directions in combination with jumping to receive a pass, intercept a ball or rebound. The sudden stop-start motion of the game is what often leads to serious injuries in participants. Higher grade players, in both senior and junior competitions, are more susceptible to injuries than lower grade players, due to the high intensity and rapid pace of the game. An injury is most commonly defined as one that has occurred while participating in sport and which led to one of the following consequences: a reduction in the amount or level of sports activity; need for medical advice or treatment; and/or adverse economic or social effects for the athlete.

Common Soft Tissue Injuries in Netball

A soft tissue injury is the damage of muscles, ligaments or tendons in the body. The most common soft tissue injuries in netball occur to the ankles, knees and hands. The main cause of these injuries is due to incorrect landing. Other factors influencing injury include; tripping, collisions with other players, being struck by the ball, over-exertion and fatigue.

Ankles

In netball the ankle joint is most susceptible to injury and accounts for 31% of the injuries sustained in the sport. A sprained ankle is a tear or complete rupture of a ligament. The most commonly injured ligament is the Anterior Talofibular Ligament. This ligament is on the outside of the ankle and injury occurs when the sole of the foot rolls inwards. A minor sprain may only need a week to recover, however severe ankle sprains can result in a player being out for 6–10 weeks.

Knees

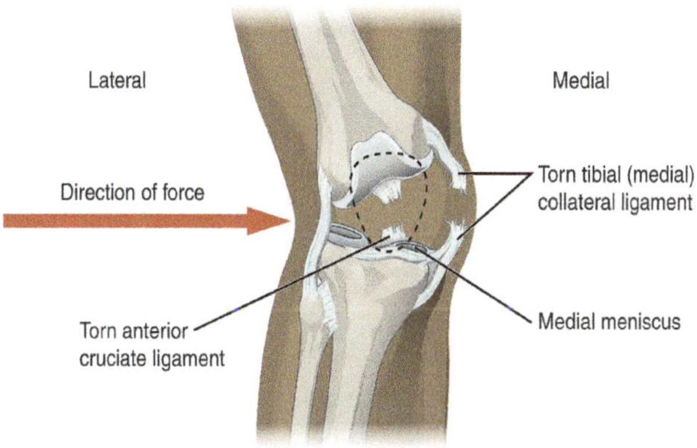

Ruptured Anterior Cruciate Ligament(ACL)

Knee injuries are the second most common injury in netball and are the most serious in regards to cost and disability. Studies show that majority of knee injuries are new injuries, and those who sustain a knee injury often withdraw from participation in netball. The most common knee injuries are meniscal and major ligament sprains/ruptures. The most commonly injured ligament is the Anterior Cruciate Ligament(ACL). The ACL allows a twisting motion at the knee. Common symptoms of an ACL rupture include a "popping" sound at the time of the injury, severe pain, swelling and a feeling of instability. ACL injuries are difficult to effectively diagnose without the assistance of Medical Resonance Imaging (MRI). A ruptured ACL will require knee reconstruction surgery that will result in the athlete being out of the game for 9–12 months.

Hands/Other

Hand injuries usually involve joint ligamentous sprains and fractures. Children most commonly injure hands, in particular their fingers. "Other" types of injuries in netball vary including; lower leg strain, quadriceps haematoma, rotator cuff shoulder problems, an elbow joint dislocation, a radial fracture, and back problems.

Treatment

As soon as an injury occurs game time must be held until the player has been properly assessed and removed from the court if need be. It is essential that players seek immediate help from a qualified first aid provider or health practitioner. Any netball injury should be treated by using the P.R.I.C.E.S., D.R.S.A.B.C., T.O.T.A.P.S. AND R.I.C.E.R. regimes:

P - Protect	D - Danger	T - Talk	R - Rest
R - Rest	R - Response	O - Observe	I - Ice
I - Ice	S - Send for help	T - Touch	C - Compression
C - Compression	A - Airway	A - Active movement	E - Elevation
E - Elevation	B - Breathing	P - Passive movement	R - Referral
S - Stabilise	C - Circulation	S - Skills test	

If an injury occurs ensure that all netball players receive adequate treatment and full rehabilitation before returning to play. Serious ankle and knee ligament ruptures will require reconstructive surgery. It is essential to follow all recovery and rehabilitation programs fully to prevent any injury from re occurring.

Netball Injury Prevention

Good Preparation

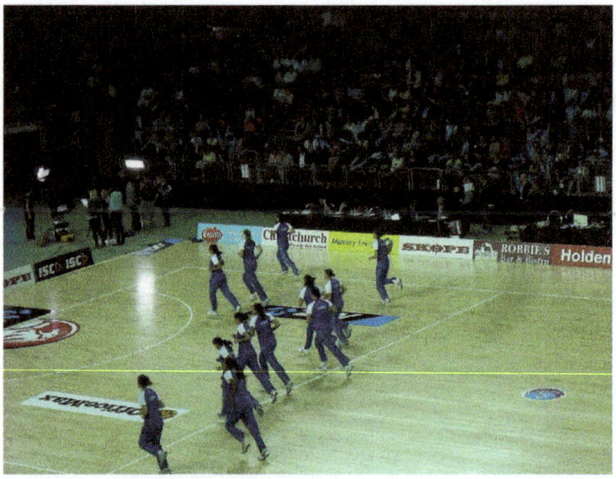

Northern Mystics warming up for their match against the Canterbury Tactix

In order to prevent netball injuries, essential pre-season training is required before commencing the playing season. The distance travelled by elite players over a game ranges from 7 km (shooters/ defenders) to 8.8 km (centre court players). A game does not only consist of basic running; players are required to accelerate in rapid bursts for the majority of the game. In pre-season training players must undertake fitness programs that focus on power, strength, agility and flexibility, especially of muscles around the ankles and feet. It is important that fitness testing is conducted prior to competition to ensure readiness to play the game.

Good Technique

Training should consist of netball specific exercises that focus on enhancing body balance, landing control, change of direction and catching passes. It is essential for coaches to undergo regular educational updates to make sure the information they have about correct training drills is current. It is very important that children are properly taught the fundamentals of netball before they participate in game situations. Any incorrect techniques should be corrected at a young age before they become a bad habit.

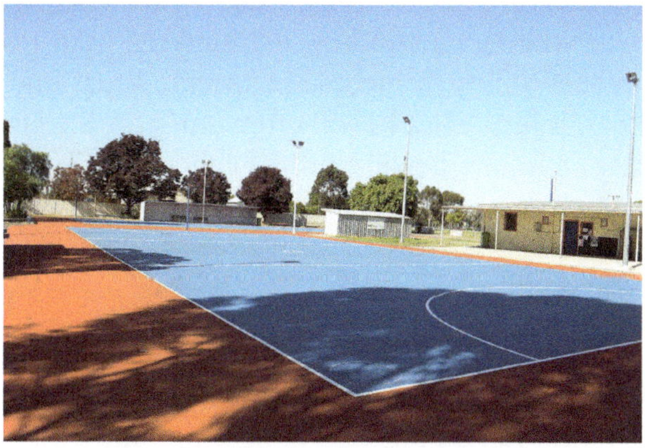

A hard but smooth netball court surface

Warm Up

A warm-up should never be overlooked in netball as it plays a vital and effective role in preventing injury. A warm-up is essential before physical activity to; prepare the body for vigorous exercise, reduce the risk of injury, reduce muscle stiffness and mentally prepare the athlete. Any warm-up should consist of running, dynamic movements and dynamic stretches. It should last for a minimum of ten minutes.

Equipment/Clothing

In netball it is essential that the goal posts are firmly fixed to the ground and have a padded post protector around them. All courts should be a firm, smooth surfaces with no loose gravel or hazards. The most important uniform item for any netball player is the shoes. It is highly recommended that players wear netball specific shoes, as they are tailored to the demands of the game and provide the correct level of support and cushioning. It is also recommended that players should wear braces or strap their ankles to provide extra support and decrease the risk of a major injury occurring.

Psychological Effects of Having a Major Injury

For many netball players a serious injury can be a traumatic life event that results in physical and psychological ramifications. The main psychological effects include the initial emotional response of experiencing an injury, the psychological factors that influence the recovery process, and the psychological impact of an injury on the athletes future performance. It is important to remember that not all injured athletes will experience the same cognitive and emotional responses.

Emotional Responses

During injury and recovery players may experience different mood states. The most commonly found mood disturbances are increases in depression, tension and anger. The emotional response will depend on how extreme the injury is. Self-efficacy is defined as one's belief in ones ability to succeed in specific situations. Physical self-efficacy is often affected by an injury. Players will often enter an extremely negative state of mind immediately after an injury, however; during recovery they often become exceedingly positive.

Self-motivation

Most often players will be highly motivated to get back to playing netball as soon as possible. However it is important to remember that injured athletes will have good and bad days. During rehabilitation an athletes motivation and enthusiasm for treatment may decrease if they are experiencing setbacks or a period of little or no improvement. It is important for athletes to have a good support network to keep them positive and focused during these harder times.

Confidence

Physical recovery is critical, however, psychological rehabilitation is the most important part of recovery. Even though a player may be physically ready to return to netball, they may not be psychologically ready to play. Various doubts, fears and anxieties may surface when thinking about returning to netball. The athlete may fear they are going to be a different player, they will not meet their coach or teammates expectations or that their physical fitness will not return to pre-injury state. This will result in the athlete putting a huge amount of pressure on themselves. This anxiety and tension can lead to the following outcomes: reinjury; injury to another body part; lowered confidence resulting in a temporary or permanent performance decrement; general depression; and fear of further injury, which can sap motivation and the desire to return to competition.

Dealing with Psychological Effects

The most successful psychological techniques that aid injury recovery are; good interpersonal communication skills, positive reinforcement, setting realistic goals, knowing methods for positive self-thoughts, coach support, and keeping the athlete involved with the team.

Returning to Pre-injury Levels & Goal Setting

Determining a successful return to netball from injury for most athletes is the ability to train and compete at pre-injury levels and standards. Measuring this includes things such as; reaching past endurance fitness test levels (beep tests); the ability to perform and complete sport-specific training exercises; and maintaining performance. Achieving these goals at training will best prepare an athlete for what they will experience during competition standards. It is important for the athlete to set realistic goals that they are able to achieve. They must understand that these goals may need to be long term, as not everything can be achieved over night. It is important that goals are flexible because when injured the rehab progress is often unpredictable.

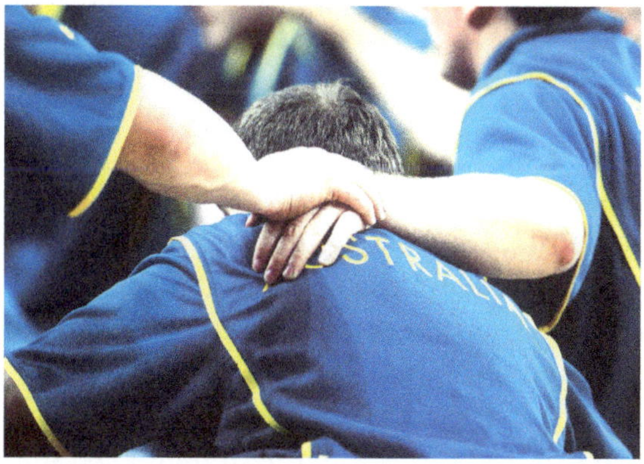

Strong support is needed from teammates, coaches, friends and family

Active Participation in Rehabilitation

Athletes that are engaged in their rehabilitation program are likely to cope with their injury more successfully. Physiotherapists state that athletes who show interest in their rehabilitation by; communicating well, asking questions, listening well to advice, and providing feedback, are more likely to have a positive psychological response to their injury.

Strong Support Systems

It is very important to have social support during the injury, rehabilitation and sports returning phase. This may include coaches, trainers, friends and family. The support of these people is essential for times when the athlete may need positive encouragement around them. The athlete should talk to someone they feel most comfortable with and who is going to listen and support them.

Sports Psychologist

It can be beneficial for an injured player to work with a sports psychologist. Coach and family can be helpful, however there may be times when they are too close to the situation and where an outside point of view is needed to help.

Take it Slow

It is important to remember that there is no rush to get back to netball. Athletes should feel prepared and confident before returning to competition. It is important to take part in game play situations at training. The athlete may also want to start in a lower grade then usual to help ease back into the game. They should aim to play one quarter in their first game back, and slowly build from there aiming to play a full game as they have progressed and experienced success.

Controversies

Hypermobility and Injuries in Junior Netball Players

Hypermobility is defined as a condition in which an individual's synovial joints have a range of motion beyond normal limits. Hypermobile joints can be a performance enhancement in some sports, for example spin bowlers in cricket. However some studies suggest the increased risk of joint dislocations, sprains and joint hyperextension in athletes with hypermobile joints. They believe that recognising hyper mobility in young female athletes may reduce the risk of injuries occurring. On the contrary, others suggest that hyper mobility is not associated with an increased incidence of injuries in junior netball players.

Serious/Career Threatening Injuries in Elite Netball Players

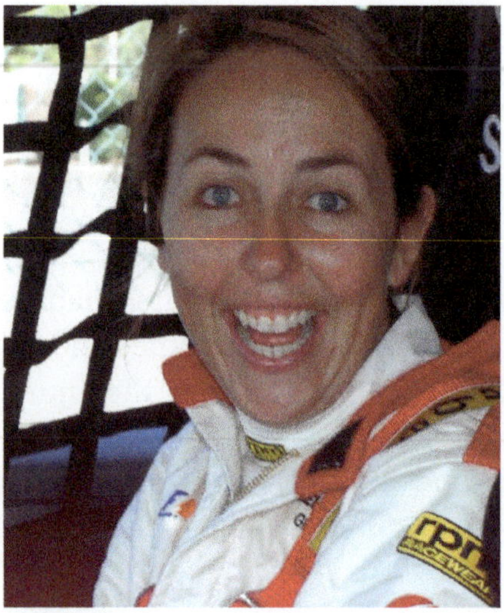

Australian netball player Liz Ellis

2005: In October 2005, Australian captain Liz Ellis, suffered a career-threatening knee injury after tearing her ACL in a match against New Zealand. This injury ruled her out of the chance to play at the 2006 Melbourne Commonwealth games. Ellis said that she had to reignite her passion and love for the game that had been her life. Ellis states that "It was soul-destroying to watch my team walk out without me and realise, hey, they can play without me".

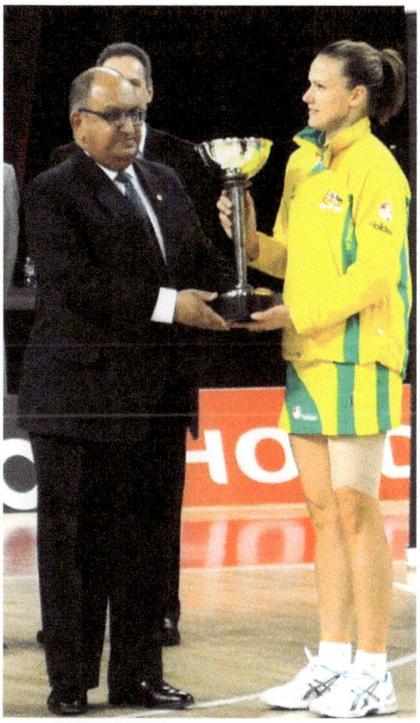

Constellation Cup Presentation 2010

She worked extremely hard on her rehabilitation, her knee repaired and her passion was restored. Ellis produced some of the best netball of her career in the two years that followed. She ended her 18-year career in her 122nd test with Australia winning the world championship 42-38. She overcame all critics and odds after coming back from her knee injury.

2012: West Coast Fever captain, Ashleigh Brazill, ruptured the meniscus in her left knee late in the 2012 ANZ championship season. Brazill had been selected to represent Australia in the Constellation Cup, but unfortunately had to withdrawal from the team. Brazil worked to build the strength back in her knee and went on to resume playing in the following 2013 season.

2014: In October 2014, KIA Magics inspirational captain, Casey Kopua suffered a knee injury during the Test of the Constellation Cup Series between Australian and New Zealand. Kopua ruptured the patella tendon in her left knee and had knee surgery to repair the tendon that would result in her missing up to 6 months of netball.

2015: In April 2015, Melbourne Vixens mid courter, Madi Robinson ruptured the anterior cruciate ligament in her right knee. Robinson missed out on the 2015 Netball World Cup. She is on track to return to play in the 2016 season.

Sports-related Traumatic Brain Injury

A sports-related traumatic brain injury is relatively uncommon, yet it is a serious accident which may lead to significant morbidity or mortality. Traumatic brain injuries (TBIs) have reduced in frequency and severity from years past due to the development of standardized rules and organized athletics. TBI in sports are usually a result of physical contact with another person or stationary object, these sports may include boxing, football, field/ice hockey, lacrosse, martial arts, rugby, soccer, wrestling, auto racing, cycling, equestrian, roller blading, skateboarding, skiing, or snowboarding.

A study was completed identifying the severity and frequency traumatic brain injuries occurred in high school sports:

"Of 23,566 reported injuries in the 10 sports during the 3-year study period, 1219 (5.5%) were MTBIs. Of the MTBIs, football accounted for 773 (63.4%) of cases; wrestling, 128 (10.5%); girls' soccer, 76 (6.2%); boys' soccer, 69 (5.7%); girls' basketball, 63 (5.2%); boys' basketball, 51 (4.2%); softball, 25 (2.1%); baseball, 15 (1.2%); field hockey, 13 (1.1%); and volleyball, 6 (0.5%). The injury rates per 100 player-seasons were 3.66 for football, 1.58 for wrestling, 1.14 for girls' soccer, 1.04 for girls' basketball, 0.92 for boys' soccer, 0.75 for boys' basketball, 0.46 for softball, 0.46 for field hockey, 0.23 for baseball, and 0.14 for volleyball. The median time lost from participation for all MTBIs was 3 days. There were 6 cases of subdural hematoma and intracranial injury reported in football. Based on these data, an estimated 62,816 cases of MTBI occur annually among high school varsity athletes participating in these sports, with football accounting for about 63% of cases."

The most common TBIs in sports are cerebral contusions, second impact syndrome concussions, dementia pugilistica, and hematomas.

Concussions

Epidemiology

A concussion is defined as a stunning, damaging, or shattering effect from a hard blow; especially: a jarring injury of the brain resulting in disturbance of cerebral function. Concussions are also sometimes referred to as mTBI (Mild Traumatic Brain Injury). Concussions are injuries to the head which cause a temporary lapse in the normal operation of brain function. Concussions have many symptoms which could be displayed in a physical, psychological or emotional manner. Concussions symptoms can sometimes be hard to determine because they present in a subtle manner. A symposium was held in 2008 in Zurich, Switzerland where a definition for concussions was developed. A concussion is now defined as "a complex pathophysiological process affecting the brain, induced by traumatic biomechanical forces."

There are five major features in conjunction with the definition:

- Concussion may be caused either by a direct blow to the head, face, or neck or elsewhere on the body with an "implosive" force transmitted to the head.
- Concussion typically results in the rapid onset of short-lived impairment of neurologic function that resolves spontaneously.
- Concussion may result in neuro-pathological changes, but the acute clinical symptoms largely reflect a functional disturbance rather than a structural injury.
- Concussion results in a graded set of clinical symptoms that may or may not involve loss of consciousness. Resolution of the clinical and cognitive symptoms typically follows a sequential course; however, it is important to note that in a small percentage of cases, post concussive symptoms may be prolonged.
- No abnormality on standard structural neuroimaging studies is seen in concussion.

Signs and Symptoms in Sports

Signs and symptoms of concussions can be hard to determine because they may not present strongly and because they may not present for several hours after the incident has occurred. There are 4 categories that symptoms of a concussion can be classified within: physical, cognitive, emotional and sleep disturbance. The most common symptom is a headache as well as the feeling of being "fog like". Other, more subtle symptoms that can accompany headaches are emotional changes, irritability, slowed reaction times and drowsiness. Accompanying symptoms can include sensitivity to light, and noise, fatigue, dizziness, nausea and vomiting. The loss of consciousness is another identifiable characteristic of concussions but it is not a required symptom to diagnose it. The loss of consciousness occurs in only 10% of concussions, so it cannot be a reliable sign of a concussion. Other distinguishing characteristics of concussions are retrograde amnesia (loss of memory just prior to injury) and posttraumatic amnesia (impaired recall of time between the injury or resumption of consciousness and the point at which new memories are stored and retrieved).

Diagnosis in Sports

There are many diagnostic tools and tests within sports. While the tests and scales may vary greatly from sport to sport, in the end, they effectively gain the same information regardless. The first initial assessment that should take place with every athlete found to be unconscious after head or neck trauma is the "ABC's" (airway, breathing, and circulation). There is an array of initial sideline evaluations that can be conducted after a possible concussive incident such as Maddocks questions, Standardized Assessment of Concussion (SAC), Balance Error Scoring System (BESS), or Sport Concussion Assessment Tool 2 (SCAT2). "The Maddocks questions are a brief set of questions to evaluate orientation as well as short and long-term memory related to the sport and current game. The questions are for sideline use only and are included in the SCAT2." The BESS test is a test based on an athlete's posture. There are 3 positions that the athlete tests in and a composite score of their errors over the 6 rounds of testing determines their scores. The SCAT2 uses both the BESS and SAC test. The SAC and SCAT-2 evaluations also contain symptoms checklists which can determine immediate cognitive and motor deficits, although many symptoms may present hours after the initial injury. 85% of certified athletic trainers use symptom checklists as part of a concussion assessment according to a recent survey.

Limited research of the test since its release from the Zurich Concussion statement has not allowed it to be verified as a successful testing method. The SAC however, does have sufficient evidence regarding it's reliability, with researchers finding the test having a test-retest reliability of 53%. Many major professional sports organizations like the NFL, NHL, MLB and NBA have taken stronger looks at in game concussions through extensive studies to develop safer equipment and playing conditions for the players. In doing this they have developed their own initial sideline testing and concussion protocols. The NFL has adopted a standardized testing evaluation form based on the SCAT2 that it has implemented into all head and neck trauma incidents. In 2011 the NFL changed their concussion protocol and built upon their previous SCAT2 standardized test. "The new implementations include a focused screening neurological examination to exclude cervical spine and intracranial bleeding, assessment of orientation, immediate and delayed recall, concentration, as well as a balance evaluation."

Similarly in 2011, the NHL adopted a new league wide concussion protocol which would remove players from the bench, who may have possibly sustained head or neck trauma, and bring them back to an undisclosed quiet room. Players would be held there for a minimum of 15 minutes while completing tests similar of those to the NFL's testing protocol. In 2007 Major League Baseball also adopted a concussion program for umpires and players. In 2011 the policy was revised and 4 new features were added to the program. The first of which is that all umpires and players are to conduct base line testing during spring training or after a player signing. Secondly, the SCAT2 has been adopted as the official sideline test for all MLB teams. Thirdly, a 7-day disabled list has been set up for players with concussions; players on the list for 14 days are moved to the 15-day disabled list. Lastly, the leagues medical director must clear all players who have suffered a concussion before they can return to play. Of the four major professional sports in the U.S., the NBA is the only league to have not adopted a sideline concussion policy. Each team and their medical staff proceed differently with their policies.

Prognosis (Short/Long-term Effects)

Short-term Effects

Short-term effects deal mostly with Post-concussion Syndrome, which has no clearly defined definition. A person suffering from a single concussive incident typically has a strong recovery rate. The most common Post-concussion symptom is a persistent headache which usually disappears within 1–2 weeks. Other common short-term effects include dizziness, vomiting, nausea, sensitivity to light and sound, irritability, cognitive lapses and memory impairment. 20-90% of the persons affected develop one symptom within a month of the incident, after 3 months 40% of the affected persons show at least 3 symptoms.

Long-term Effects

Receiving multiple concussive incidents has long been known to cause a cumulative effect on the brain. It is also known that each successive concussion makes it easier to obtain another concussion in the future. Receiving multiple concussions can lead to long-term memory loss, psychiatric disorders, brain damage and other neurological disorders. There are no clearly defined guidelines for the retirement of an athlete, but it has been proposed that an athlete who sustains 3 concussive incidents in a single season or has Post-concussion symptoms for more than 3 months should consider a lengthy period away from the sport. Especially with sports, when multiple concussions are received it is likely that a doctor will advise the player in question to avoid returning to sports where contact is possible.

Second-impact Syndrome

Second-impact syndrome (SIS) occurs when an athlete sustains a second concussive incident before the symptoms of a prior concussive incident have fully healed. It does not take a severe concussion to cause SIS, even a mild grade concussion can lead to it. The condition is often fatal, and if death does not occur severe disability is probable. SIS is most often developed in young athletes, who are thought to be particularly vulnerable.

Prevention in Sports

Helmets

Throughout the progression of contact sports there have been continual innovations in protective gear, especially in terms of limiting head and neck traumas. The earliest known use of football helmets is documented in an 1893 Army-Navy game. Early helmets were typically only constructed of leather padding. Throughout the early 1900s helmets developed to include metal and plastics to better protect the player. In 1939 helmets became mandatory for college players, and a year later the NFL adopted the same policy. The increasing development and standardization of helmets along with rule changes that would protect players, would eventually cut down on head and neck traumas. In 2012 testing is being conducted on a new type of helmet which battles rotational acceleration which is linked closer to concussions than typical impacts. This helmet is called the Multidirectional Impact Protection System (MIPS). This new generation of helmet is shown to decrease rotational acceleration by 55% compared to the traditional football helmet. Like the NFL the NHL took steps to protecting players by mandating helmets in 1979. As of 2009 about 60% of NHL players currently wear a half visor for upper face protection.

Mouth Guards

Many sports including football, ice hockey, lacrosse, field hockey, and boxing implemented mandatory mouth guard policies during the 1960s and 70's. These policies were introduced to cut down on a player's chance of orofacial injury and concussions. Several studies conducted in many various professional and collegiate sports have yet to validate the claim that mouth guards cut down on concussions; although a study conducted by the NHL showed that symptom severity had significantly decreased with the use of mouth guards.

Cerebral Contusions

Epidemiology

Cerebral contusions are bruises to the brain caused by a direct blow to the head causing the brain to bounce against the inside of the skull and bruise brain tissue. The force of the blow causes either a tearing or twisting of the structure and blood vessels which hinders the ability of the receptors to send feedback to the brain. With the tearing or twisting of structure, the brain begins to swell and bleed. Since the brain cavity has no room to expand due to the swelling, bruises begin to form. Due to the nature of the injury, most of the contusive damage is found deeper in the brain.

In sports, most cerebral contusions are caused when the brain is either suddenly accelerated, decelerated, or strikes an immovable object. When the blow happens, brain tissue can be damaged, sometimes resulting in the need for hospitalization and surgery. A resection of the contused tissue is needed within surgery pending the severity of the incident. The highest rates of contusions occur in men between the ages of 15 to 24, somewhat due to their aggressive nature. If a person sustains a contusion one time, they are more likely to sustain a repeated one.

Signs and Symptoms in Sports

In the heat of a game, it may be hard to see or feel symptoms relating to cerebral contusions. If any of these signs are visible or as an athlete, you feel them, remove yourself from competition immediately. Cerebral contusions and other injuries can occur in any sport, not just in the traditional "collision" sports. According to the US-CPSC, four of the top five sports that cause brain injuries are considered to have limited brain contact: basketball, bicycling, baseball, and playground activities. The most popular sport to cause cerebral contusions is American football due to the drastic acceleration/deceleration of the brain.

Immediate Signs of a Cerebral Contusion

- Headache
- Nausea
- Slurred speech
- Restlessness
- Pupil dilation
- Memory loss
- Personality shift
- Seizures

Post-game Symptoms

- Loss of consciousness
- Severe headaches
- Coma (due to loss of consciousness)

If any of these symptoms are felt or noticed, a hospital visit is needed where further machine testing is done. In boxing, the rapid deceleration of the brain after an impact causes the symptoms to progress much faster or at a more traumatic rate. Doctors ringside monitor a boxer's attitude and brain function throughout the fight and are able to stop the match following startling news.

Diagnosis in Sports

Contusions are identified with two forms of diagnosis: acceleration of the brain and direct trauma. A direct trauma injury is much more severe than an acceleration injury (in most cases) and requires much more intensive diagnosis and testing. The full extent of the injury may not be known until testing done in a hospital is complete.

In football, medical trainers are well versed to diagnose symptoms pertaining to a traumatic brain injury. They are not, however, able to determine what type of injury it is or the extent the injury stems. Football trainers can medically clear or not clear players based on brain injury symptoms. If a trainer feels that certain symptoms exist that are similar to that of cerebral contusions, they will take the player out of the game and rush them to the hospital. Upon admission into the hospital, a CT scan will be ordered. A CT scan is the quickest method to diagnose cerebral contusions because it can be performed immediately and have fairly exact findings. The best method, as suggested by medical doctors, is an MRI because they present more sensitive and accurate findings. MRI's, however, must be scheduled and cannot be completed immediately following the injury. MRI's also take a long time to perform where the injury a player sustained may get worse within that time frame.

Case Study Example

History: The individual is possibly unconscious when examined by medical personnel on the field. A common symptom is prolonged unconsciousness (coma), however this player reports headache, dizziness, nausea, vomiting, and weakness of the extremities (paresis) and makes inappropriate responses to questions.

Physical exam: The individual's level of consciousness is disturbed. A neurological examination may not reveal any localizing signs. The individual with no other serious injuries than cerebral contusion will not have a fractured skull or any signs of opening or penetration of the skull.

Tests: Skull x-rays check for a fracture. CT or MRI detect any bleeding in the skull. The Glasgow Coma Scale classifies the severity of brain injury, with a score of 15 as normal and progressively lower scores indicating greater neurologic injury to the brain.

After testing is completed, doctors will make an estimate on the extent of the injury and possible recovery time. If cranial bleeding and swelling is minor, a short hospital stay (up to a week) is needed with close observation. If bleeding is severe, the player may be treated as a patient with a severe head injury (with surgery as the main option). This process requires the patient to be admitted into an intinsive care unity with close monitoring of blood levels and brain activity.

Prognosis (Short/Long-term Effects)

The effects of a cerebral contusion depend on the cause of the injury and what part of the brain was most affected. Outcomes vary from minor injuries that require short recovery times to severe injuries that can lead to death. Short-term effects of cerebral contusions can range from a mild headache to feeling lightheaded for a few days. Most short-term effects match that of a mild head injury while long-term effects can be much more serious. Most long-term injuries require surgery, rehabilitation, and close monitoring. In small cases, cerebral contusions can lead to death (about 15 per 100,000 people). If a cerebral contusion leads to a coma, recovery can be very long and rehabilitation extensive. If the coma is long, the probability of dying or permanent neurological damage is very possible.

Prevention in Sports

Rules exist within each sport to help prevent cerebral contusions and traumatic brain injuries. However, individual athletes are the best prevention against their own injuries. In a game, athletes notice when they have the symptoms of a cerebral contusion and should take themselves out of the game. It may be hard for medical personnel or coaches to notice when a player has a traumatic brain injury, so it is in the player's best interest to be removed from play. In hockey, traumatic brain injuries constitute 10%-15% of all head injuries. With the high percent of injuries being traumatic, extensive design improvements have been made to helmets. These improvements reduce the risk of cerebral contusions by providing more padding around the skull and a chin strap that keeps the helmet snug. In baseball, major improvements to helmets have been made to protect batters from the impact a baseball can have when hitting their head. Helmets, before this major improvement, were designed to withstand a velocity of 70 mph from a pitch or foul ball. Since the company Rawlings' new design, helmets can withstand a velocity of 100 mph and have further padding around the softer parts on the side of the skull.

Dementia Pugilistica (Punch-drunk Syndrome)

Epidemiology

A syndrome affecting boxers that is caused by cumulative cerebral injuries and is characterized by impaired cognitive processes (as thinking and remembering), Parkinsonism, impaired and often slurred speech, and slow poorly coordinated movements especially of the legs. Dementia Pugilistica, more commonly known as "Punch Drunk Syndrome", is a degenerative brain disorder resulting from head trauma. Dementia Pugilistica (DP) is typically associated with the sport of boxing; although symptoms of DP may appear immediately after a single traumatic brain injury, they are typically described following the cessation of exposure to chronic brain injury.

Signs and Symptoms in Sports

Some of the subjective symptoms experienced after a Knockout are headaches, tinnitus, forgetfulness, impaired hearing, dizziness, nausea and impaired gait. Approximately ten percent of these active boxers reported constantly suffering from forgetfulness, headaches and other symptoms. Symptoms can be progressive and can develop late into a boxer's career or possibly years into retirement. Some of the earlier symptoms of "punch drunk syndrome" are noticeable in extremities; such as trembling hands or feet, or an instability in equilibrium. Signs of chronic brain damage can also affect irritability, paranoia and cause violent outbursts.

Diagnosis in Sports

Dementia pugilistica is difficult to diagnose until the later stages of a boxer's life. Symptoms are not apparent until boxer's are years into retirement. The damage is done in four primary sites of the brain: the septal regions, the cerebellum, the substantia nigra and the neurons. The septa end up separated and torn apart while the ventricles become enlarged. "The main motor pathways in the cerebellum and substantia nigra are affected, as well as the foramen magnum." Lastly, the neurons in the brains of boxer's have a "bizarre tendency for many neurons, mainly in the deep temporal grey matter, to develop abnormal neurofibrils called Alzheimer tangle. The most successful way to diagnose DP is through magnetic resonance imaging techniques, more commonly known as an MRI. Segmented inversion recovery ratio imaging technique is based on the ratio of a white matter suppressed image and gray matter suppressed image. "The (SIRRIM) technique improves the differentiation of gray matter from white matter and is sensitive to detect abnormalities of intracellular space, including changes during cellular death."

Prognosis (Short/Long-term Effects)

Multiple studies have concluded that there is neurological evidence of damage to pyramidal, extrapyramidal and cerebellar systems with associated psychosis, memory loss or dementia, personality change and social instability. After fighting, boxers show raised levels of brain chemicals neurofilament light protein and total tau then they did after three months with no boxing.

Prevention in Sports

Protective measures have been taken especially in amateur boxing, such as the wearing of a head guard, more heavily cushioned gloves (weighing 10 ounces in amateur boxing and 8 ounces in professional boxing), shorter and fewer rounds, the addition of the 'outclassed rule' (where the point difference becomes greater than 20), and the option for the boxer to interrupt the fight itself.

Hematoma

Epidemiology

A hematoma is a localized collection of blood that gathers outside the blood vessels in an area it does not belong. Specifically a hematoma is tissue damage due to acceleration or deceleration from unrestricted movement, in which the result is shearing of the brain tissue. Two types of hematomas occurring within the brain are: subdural and extradural hematomas, which are classified as a traumatic brain injury (TBI). When a direct blow to the head occurs, there is bruising to the brain and damage to the internal tissue and blood vessels. Additionally, the jarring of the brain against the skull causes hematomas. Injuries commonly occur during contact sport such as boxing, football, basketball, motor cycling, scuba diving, mountaineering, hang gliding, skydiving, and horseback riding. Council on scientific affairs. Following a serve brain injury or a skull fracture one of the two hematomas may occur. An extradural hematoma is a TBI where blood collects between the inside of the skull and the dura, the thick outer covering of the brain. A subdural hematoma is when a localized collection of blood occurs under the surface of the dura matter. Blood collects on the outermost layer of the brain and creates an intracranial pressure.

Signs and Symptoms in Sports

Generally, symptoms for hematomas are confused speech, difficulty with balance or walking, headaches, lethargy or confusion, nausea or vomiting, numbness, seizures, slurred speech, visual disturbances, and weakness. For example, an athlete who experiences a subdural hematoma will experience loss of consciousness with little or no lucidity. Pupils are often dilated or unequal. Additionally, hemiparesis, seizure activity, and vomiting, may be apparent. An epidural hematoma typically results in serve a headache which is followed by a brief loss of consciousness and variable levels of lucidness. This may last for several hours while the brain function deteriorates. If untreated epidural hematoma causes increased blood pressure, shortness of breath, damage to brain function and may result in death.

Diagnosis in Sports

Subdural and epidural hematomas are serious conditions and should be immediately diagnosed and treated by a physician. Hematomas may not show the full extent of the problem initially after the head injury, but it may be revealed after comprehensive medical evaluation and diagnostic test. Diagnostic test may include: blood test, x-ray, computed tomography scan (CT/CAT scan), electroencephalogram (EEG), and magnetic resonance imaging (MRI). The two most important diagnostic tests are the CT scan and the MRI. The CT scan reveals evidence of blood within the skull, fractures, and signs of compression on the brain from the hematoma. The MRI is a more thorough evaluation of injuries to the brain tissue. Yet, a MRI cannot take place if the injured victim is in a confused state. Small hematomas may not require surgery if there is no pressure on the brain and minimal symptoms. Small hematomas may be monitored closely to ensure the hematoma is not enlarging and resolved properly. A large hematoma larger than 1 cm at its thickest point produces severe headaches and brain function deterioration requires immediate surgery by a neurosurgeon. Surgery reduces the pressure within the brain and stops the bleeding.

Prognosis (Short/Long-term Effects)

The most crutial aspect for recovery in patients with severe hematomas is rapid diagnosis and appropriate treatment. Once the clot has been removed the intracranial pressure is monitored for several days. Conditions which are also monitored after surgery are seizures, clot accumulation, and infection. If complications do occur, sometime the hematoma needs to be re-drained. Additional complications following a surgical or nonsurgical treatment may include temporary or permanent weakness, numbness, difficulty speaking, memory loss, dizziness, headache, anxiety, difficulty concentrating, seizures, and/or brain herniation. The most helpful predictors of the treatment outcome is the glasgow coma scale (GCS). This is a standardized pupil response assessment of the neurologic status of the patient. GCS helps assess many different types of head injuries and predicts how a patient will recover following a hematoma. Factors such as elevated intracranial pressure, increased patients age, and abnormal GCS results lead to a poor prognosis. The mortality rate following a hematoma could be as high as 80% and survivors many not regain the same pre-injury function. Subdural and epidural hematomas are serious injuries and recovery varies widely depending on the severity of the hematoma. Severity depends on type and location of the injury, the size of the blood collection, and how quickly treatment is obtained. Hence, it is difficult to determine when an athlete can return to sports after his/her injury. A variety of multidisciplinary people such as sports medicine physicians, neurologist/neurosurgeons, athletic trainers, coaches, and family require input. If an athlete is approved to return, he or she is required to complete asymptomatic at rest and with exertion. The athlete also has to clear a CT scan indicating the hematoma has entirely resolved. Lastly, the athlete needs to be slowly brought back into the sport with close monitoring to be sure the symptoms do not recur.

Prevention in Sports

Preemptive measures include using safety equipment to reduce your risk of a head injury. Equipment examples are hard hats, bicycle or motorcycle helmets, and seat belts. To reduce the risk of hematomas, factors to avoid are taking anticoagulant medication (blood thinners, such as aspirin), long-term abuse of alcohol, repeated falls, and reoccurring head injury.

Second-impact Syndrome

Second-impact syndrome (SIS) occurs when the brain swells rapidly, and catastrophically, after a person suffers a second concussion before symptoms from an earlier one have subsided. This second blow may occur minutes, days or weeks after an initial concussion, and even the mildest grade of concussion can lead to SIS. The condition is often fatal, and almost everyone who is not killed is severely disabled. The cause of SIS is uncertain, but it is thought that the brain's arterioles lose their ability to regulate their diameter, and therefore lose control over cerebral blood flow, causing massive cerebral edema.

Most cases of SIS have occurred in young people, who are thought to be particularly vulnerable. In order to prevent SIS, guidelines have been established to prohibit athletes from returning to a game prematurely. For example, professionals recommend that athletes not return to play before symptoms of an initial head injury have resolved.

Due to the very small number of recorded cases of SIS, there is doubt about whether it is a valid diagnosis. However, the syndrome is recognized by physicians.

Epidemiology

Though the incidence of second impact syndrome is unknown, the condition is rare; very few cases have been confirmed in medical literature. In the 13-year period from

1980–1993, 35 American football related cases of SIS were recorded, but only 17 of these were confirmed by necropsy or surgery and magnetic resonance imaging to be due to SIS, and 18 cases were found to be probably SIS-related. Additionally, the initial trauma commonly goes unreported, adding to the confusion about how often the syndrome occurs.

By one estimate, the syndrome kills four to six people under the age of 18 per year. According to the Centers for Disease Control, about 1.5 people die each year from concussion in the US; in most of these cases, the person had received another concussion previously.

In part due to the poor documentation of the initial injury and continuing symptoms in recorded cases, some professionals think that the condition is over-diagnosed, and some doubt the validity of the diagnosis altogether.

Risks

Second-impact syndrome shares all the risk factors of concussion; that is, those who are at increased risk for concussion are also at higher risk for SIS. Thus, people who participate in sports such as boxing, soccer, American football, baseball, rugby, basketball, ice hockey, pro wrestling, and skiing (especially Alpine) are at increased risk. The condition most commonly occurs in American football.

Second-impact syndrome disproportionately affects teenagers. All documented cases occurred in people younger than 20 except in boxing. As of 2000, the syndrome had never been reported in the medical literature in children younger than adolescent age. Young athletes have been found to be both more susceptible to concussions and more likely to get second-impact syndrome than their older counterparts. However, SIS is also a concern for adult athletes. Adolescent and young adult males who play American football or hockey, or who box or ski are the most common sufferers of the condition. Every documented case of SIS has occurred in males, but it is not known whether this is due to a special vulnerability or to a greater exposure of males to second impacts.

Studies have found that people who have received one concussion are at a higher risk to receive a concussion in the future.

Features

SIS is the most serious potential complication that could result from an athlete returning to a game before symptoms from a minor head injury have subsided. Such symptoms include headache, cognitive difficulties, or visual changes.

The initial injury may be a concussion, or it may be another, more severe, type of head trauma, such as cerebral contusion. However, the first concussion need not be severe for the second impact to cause SIS. Also, the second impact may be very minor, even a blow such as an impact to the chest that causes the head to jerk, thereby transmitting forces of acceleration to the brain. Loss of consciousness during the second injury is not necessary for SIS to occur. Both injuries may take place in the same game.

The athlete may continue playing in the game after the second concussion, and may walk off the field without assistance, but symptoms quickly progress and the condition can rapidly worsen. Neurological collapse can occur within a short period, with rapid onset of dilating pupils, loss of eye movement, unconsciousness, and respiratory failure. Failure of the brain stem frequently occurs between two and five minutes after the second impact, and death can follow shortly.

SIS is sometimes associated with a small subdural hematoma.

Pathophysiology

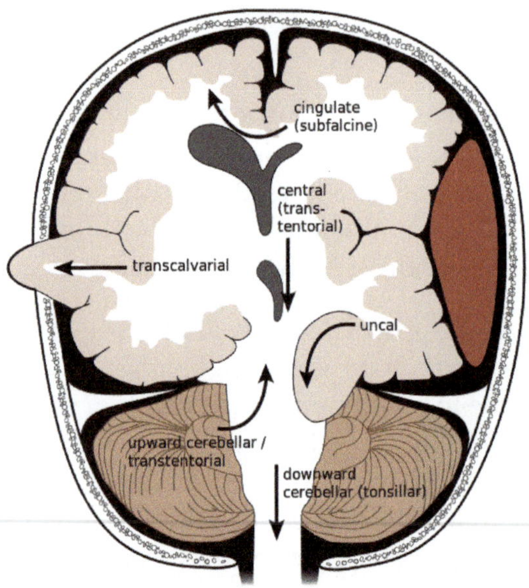

Types of brain herniation 1) Uncal 2) Central - *The brainstem herniates caudally.* 3) Cingulate herniation - *The brain squeezes under the falx cerebri.* 4) Transcalvarial herniation - *through a skull fracture* 5) Upward herniation *of the cerebellum* 6) Tonsillar herniation - *the cerebellar tonsils herniate through the foramen magnum.*

Concussion temporarily changes the brain's function. It is believed that the brain is left in a vulnerable state after concussion and that a second blow is linked to SIS. The actual mechanism behind the catastrophic brain swelling is controversial. A second injury during this time is thought to unleash a series of metabolic events within the brain. Changes indicative of SIS may begin occurring in the injured brain within 15 seconds of the second concussion. Pathophysiological changes in SIS can include a loss of autoregulation of the brain's blood vessels, which causes them to become congested. The vessels dilate, greatly increasing their diameter and leading to a large increase in cerebral blood flow. Progressive cerebral edema may also occur. The increase of blood and brain volume within the skull causes a rapid and severe increase in intracranial pressure, which can in turn cause uncal and cerebellar brain herniation, a disastrous and potentially fatal condition in which the brain is squeezed past structures within the skull.

Studies on animals have shown that the brain may be more vulnerable to a second concussive injury administered shortly after a first. In one such study, a mild impact administered within 24 hours of another one with minimal neurological impairment caused massive breakdown of the blood brain barrier and subsequent brain swelling. Loss of this protective barrier could be responsible for the edema found in SIS.

Animal studies have shown that the immature brain may be more vulnerable to brain trauma; these findings may provide clues as to why SIS affects only people under age 18.

Prevention

Measures that prevent head injuries in general also prevent SIS. Thus athletes are advised to use protective gear such as helmets, though helmets do not entirely prevent the syndrome.

Experts advise that athletes who have suffered one concussion and still complain of concussion-related symptoms be prohibited from returning to the game due to the possibility of developing SIS. Athletes are also discouraged from returning to play until after they have been evaluated and approved for resuming the sport by a healthcare provider skilled in evaluating concussion. Some athletes may deny concussion symptoms because they do not wish to be prevented from rejoining the game. Thus athletic trainers may prohibit return to play for any athlete who has suffered a concussion, regardless of the speed with which the symptoms reportedly resolve. An initial head injury may impair an athlete's judgment and ability to decide to refrain from participating in risky activity, so some healthcare providers encourage family members and other acquaintances to pressure an athlete not to return to play.

Several different sets of return-to-play guidelines exist for athletes who have suffered minor head trauma. These exist in part to prevent the player from developing SIS. A variety of concussion grading systems have been devised, in part to aid in this determination. Every return-to-play guideline recommends that an athlete not return to competition until all concussion symptoms are absent during both rest and exercise. The American Academy of Neurology recommends that young athletes be prohibited from returning to play for at least a week in most cases of concussion.

The current return-to-play guidelines may not be strict enough to protect young athletes from SIS. On the other hand, they may be too strict for professional football players; evidence that the syndrome exists in this population is lacking.

Diagnosis

Magnetic resonance imaging and computed tomography are the most useful imaging tools for detecting SIS. The congestion in the brain's blood vessels may be visible using CT scans.

SIS is distinct from repetitive head injury syndrome, in which a person suffers a series of minor head injuries over time and experiences a slow decline in functions such as cognitive abilities. Unlike SIS, repetitive head injury syndrome may still occur even when symptoms from prior injuries have completely resolved. SIS is thought to be more severe than repetitive head injury syndrome in both the short- and long-term.

Treatment

Treatment of the loss of autoregulation of the brain's blood vessels may be difficult or impossible. When SIS occurs, surgery does not help and there is little hope for recovery. Treatment requires immediate recognition and includes administration of osmotic agents and hyperventilation in order to lower intracranial pressure.

Prognosis

The mortality rate for SIS approaches 50%, and morbidity (disability) is almost 100%. Since the condition is so rare, the connection between SIS and future disability has been difficult to establish and is therefore poorly understood.

When SIS is not fatal, the effects similar to those of severe traumatic brain injury can occur, including persistent muscle spasms and tenseness, emotional instability, hallucinations, post-traumatic epilepsy, mental disability, paralysis, coma, and brain death.

History

The condition was first described in 1973 by R.C. Schneider, and the term second-impact syndrome was coined in 1984. In 1984, R.L. Saunders described the death of a football player who had died after a second, unremarkable concussion and hypothesized that the second blow caused a catastrophic rise in ICP, possibly through loss of vasomotor tone, because the brain was in a vulnerable state. Between 1984 and 1991, only four cases were documented. Between 1992 and 1998, reports of the condition began to be made more frequently than they had before, a fact is thought to be due to wider recognition of the syndrome by clinicians. In 1991, J.P. Kelly and others reported another football death after repeated concussions and coined the term "vascular congestion syndrome".

In 2002, a high-school football player from Texas named Will Benson suffered two concussions within two weeks; he collapsed shortly after the second one and died six days later as the result. He is thought to have died from SIS. Will's Bill, a law for which the father of the player had advocated after his death, was passed in Texas in June 2007. The law mandates basic emergency and safety training for sports officials in high schools, including education about second-impact syndrome, with a special focus on concussion symptoms.

In 2005, Preston Plevretes, a football player for LaSalle University, had his life changed forever by second-impact syndrome. After undergoing a head-to-head hit at football practice, a university doctor diagnosed Plevretes with a concussion and two days later was told he was allowed to resume play. Three games after returning Plevretes sustained another concussion resulting in second-impact syndrome. He was rushed to the hospital where doctors cut the right side of his skull. Five years after the injury, he still struggles to do everyday activities. Because of Plevretes, the NCAA revised concussion guidelines. The NCAA strongly urges schools to have a concussion management plan. They also require that an athlete have clearance by a team doctor before being allowed to return.

In 2006, Zachary Lystedt, a thirteen-year-old football player, suffered a concussion during one of his games. He shrugged off the hit and went back in the game a few plays later. At the end of the game, he collapsed on the field. Lystedt had second-impact syndrome. He was airlifted to a hospital where surgeons cut both sides of his skull so that the blood clot could be taken out. He was in the hospital for months and he still has trouble doing everyday things, such as walking. To prevent other families from going through what they went through, the Lystedt family made it their goal to make a law that athletes who are suspected of a concussion are not allowed to return to play unless he or she is cleared by a licensed physician. The law is now effective in over thirty states.

By 2003, 21 cases of SIS had been reported in medical literature.

Controversy

The existence of SIS is in question and is somewhat controversial. The sudden collapse seen in sufferers may be due to a type of cerebral edema that can follow an initial impact in children and teenagers, rather than to SIS. This type of edema, referred to as *diffuse cerebral swelling*, may be the real reason for the collapse which young people sometimes experience and which is commonly thought to be due to SIS. Those who doubt the validity of the diagnosis cite the finding that diffuse cerebral swelling is more common in children and adolescents as an explanation for the greater frequency of SIS diagnoses in young people. One group found that of 17 previously identified cases of SIS, only 5 met their diagnostic criteria for the syndrome, with some cases not clearly involving a second impact. They found that diagnoses of SIS were frequently based on bystander accounts of previous injuries, which they showed to be unreliable. Teammates of players who are thought to have SIS may over-report the initial concussion, giving the appearance of a greater number of second impacts than actually exist. Thus critics argue that the small number of reported cases leaves the question of whether SIS really causes the brain to swell catastrophically unanswered.

Whether a second impact is really involved in the diffuse cerebral swelling that occurs on rare occasions after a mild traumatic brain injury is controversial, but some experts agree that such catastrophic brain swelling does occur after a very small number of mild brain injuries and that young age is associated with increased risk. It is also agreed that some people may be particularly vulnerable to catastrophic brain swelling as the result of multiple head injuries.

Swimming Injuries

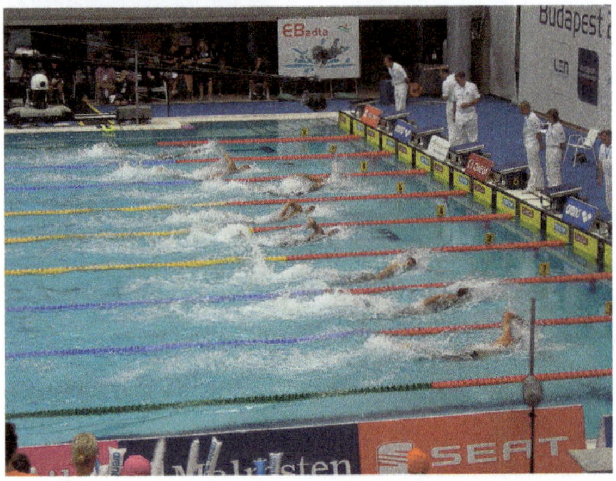

Swimming injuries have many different causes, which can occur immediate or can occur as the result of a long-term swimming career. Some ways that swimmers can increase the risk of an injury are by overuse of a specific part of the body, lacking crucial flexibility and strength, etc. These injuries, like swimmer's shoulder and breaststroker's knee, cause pain to the swimmer in certain regions that permit necessary movement for the required precise technique. Although these injuries can halt a professional swimmer's career, many can be treated and some can even be prevented. There are different procedures and exercises that can either prevent an injury or help with recovering from an injury. Many of the exercises are specific to the injury and vary in helpfulness according to the person and the technique used for the exercise.

Swimmer's Shoulder

Swimmers shoulder is the name given to a broad range of shoulder injuries that occur in swimmers and results in pain felt within the shoulder and in areas surrounding the shoulder, including down the arm and up the neck. Pain associated with swimmers shoulder often starts as an irritating niggle when swim training and can persist to intense pain while swim training and also a constant pain while resting.

While there are a number of contributing factor leading to the development of swimmers shoulder, it is believed that the two main causes of swimmers shoulder are overuse and the biomechanics of the stroke also known as stroke technique.

The first cause of swimmers shoulder is overuse. Overuse of the shoulder muscles and surrounding muscles can lead to fatigue of the muscles. Due to the muscles being fatigued they are in a weakened state and with continuous use will therefore work less effectively when swimming and will result in the swimmer having to work the shoulder muscles twice as hard by taking double the amount of strokes they would usually take in order to cover the same distance. This would ultimately result in more fatigue and inflammation of the muscles. Unilateral breathing may also cause swimmers shoulder due to the fact that the opposite shoulder to the breathing arm has to work harder to support balanced position and forward movement while the head is turned. Some training equipment such as paddles and kick boards can also put stress on the shoulder and surrounding muscles and cause fatigue and inflammation.

The second cause of swimmer shoulder is the biomechanics of the stroke also known as stroke technique. Incorrect stroke technique for example the swimmers hand entering the water across the mid-line of the swimmers body then proceeding to stroke back or the swimmers hand entering the water palm out thumb down and any other type of incorrect technique when done repetitively can cause pain, fatigue and inflammation of the shoulder and surrounding muscles.

Treatment Methods

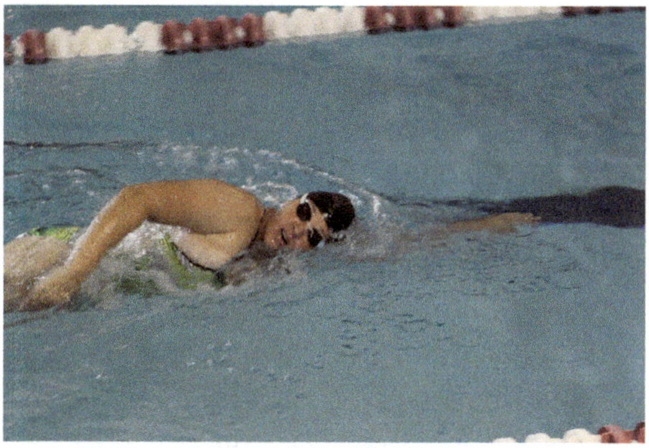

Some treatment methods include; warming up slowly prior to training, avoiding strokes & positions that cause pain (butterfly/freestyle), fixing any bad technique that could be causing the pain, adjusting the distance and frequency of training to avoid further overuse of the muscles, discontinue the use of paddles, increase kick sets to allow the shoulder to rest however limit the use of kickboards and avoid pulling sets. Increase the use of fins to assist with maintaining a good body position and to avoid drag, avoid dry land upper body weight training, ice the shoulder daily, consider the use of anti-inflammatory creams and medicines and seek the advice of a medical professional.

Breastroker's Knee

Breastroker's knee is the name given to pain felt within and around the knee that is experienced by swimmers. It is named this due to the fact it is most commonly only breastrokers that experience pain within the knee and around the knee. Most swimmer will have no problems with their knees however 'the majority (86%) of breaststroke swimmers will have experienced knee pain at one point in their career and 47.2% of them will have had this problem at least one time every week.'

There are several factors that increase the swimmers chances of developing knee pain and inflammation of the knee muscles such as, the increasing age of the swimmer, the length of the competitive career, the length of the event, inadequate warm-up, strength imbalance of hip abductors/adductors and flexibility imbalance of hip abductors/adductors.

Prevention and Treatment

In order to prevent the development of knee pain and inflammation of the knee muscles it is recommended that swimmers use a well-designed strength and stretching program, warm-up adequately, use correct breastroke kick technique, gradually build up the distance of breastroke swimming and have a balanced training program that focuses on not only breastroke and also has training sessions that allows for adequate recovery of the knee muscles to prevent fatigue of the muscles causing overuse, inflammation and pain.

Treatment of breastroker's knee includes resting the knee muscles, icing daily, elevating the limb, strengthening and stretching, support e.g. strapping or knee braces, seeking medical advice which can lead to physiotherapy, cortisone injections and in few cases surgery.

Volleyball Injuries

Volleyball is a game played between two opposing sides, with six players on each team, where the players use mainly their hands to hit the ball over a net and try to make the ball land on the opposing team's side of the court. Volleyball is played by over 800 million people world wide, making it one of the most popular sports in the world. Volleyball has some risks involved with it because there are some injuries which occur to players that are quite common; these include ankle injuries, shoulder injuries, foot injuries and knee injuries.

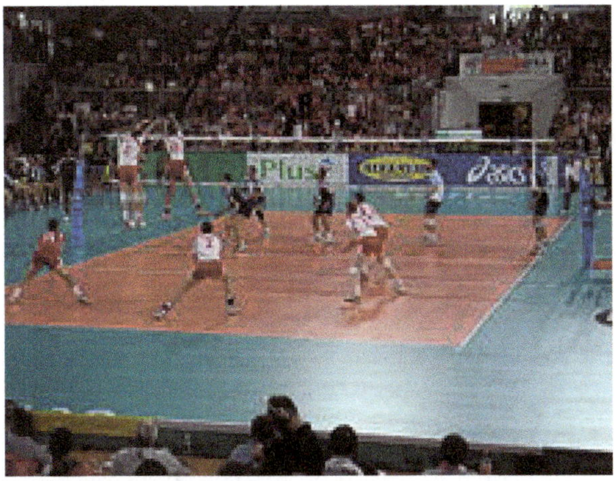

A volleyball match between Poland and Argentina

Ankle Sprains

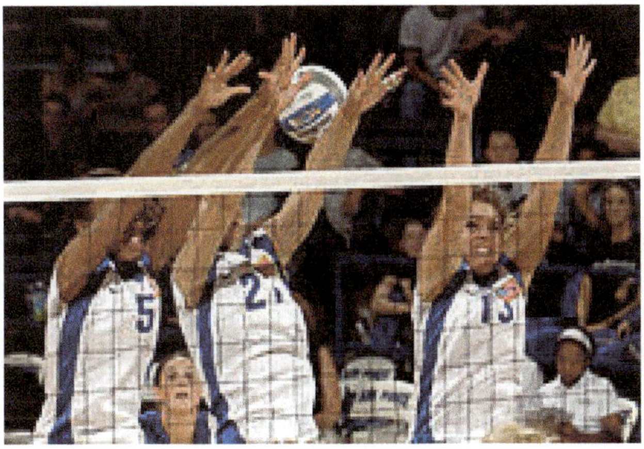

Three teammates who are attempting to block a ball have a greater risk of landing on each other's feet and spraining their ankle

The Majority of sprained ankles in volleyball occur when a player is at the net, either blocking or Spiking. The reason why ankle sprains occur at the net is because both blocking and spiking involve jumping and possibly of landing on an opponents foot causing the injury. Approximately 50 percent of all sprained ankles in volleyball occur when a blocker lands on the attacking players foot, while about 25 percent occur when a blocker lands on their own teammates foot following a block with multiple blockers involved.

One possible situation that has the possibility to cause a player to sprain their ankle is when the ball is set too tight or close to the net. As the ball is to close to the net the player who is attempting to spike the ball has to jump closer to the net meaning that they have a higher possibility of landing on or over the center line on the court. By doing this both the blockers and attacker are at an increased risk of spraining their ankle.

There are some simple ways in which ankle sprains can be prevented, which include rule changes, technical training and strapping or bracing the ankle.

Shoulder Injuries

There is currently a high number of shoulder injuries in volleyball and it is still unknown to how this number can be managed. Shoulder injuries are great in number because the shoulder is constantly placed under stress during the spiking movements and can often result in injuries to the shoulder. The stress is caused by the rotating of the arm around the shoulder joint at a high velocity. There are however multiple spiking techniques, including traditional and alternative techniques, that have different risks to the shoulder. The alternative spiking method is said to be a possible prevention to some injuries that occur in the shoulder and also enhance an athletes performance.

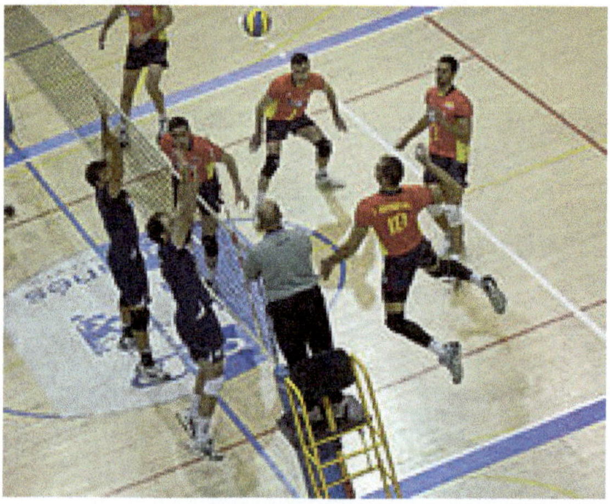

Spiking in volleyball places the shoulder under stress and can result in injury to the shoulder

Jumper's Knee

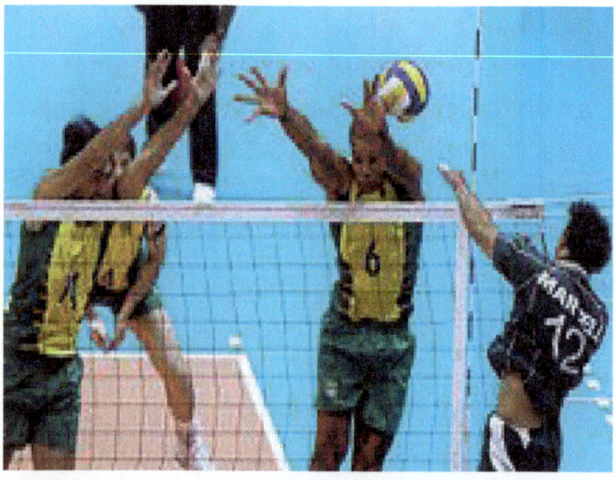

Both blocking and spiking involve jumping and have the possibility to cause Jumper's knee

Jumper's knee is injury term used in volleyball circles that describes the mechanism of the injury known as patella tendinopathy, patella tendinosis or patella tendonitis. Jumper's knee is defined as a syndrome of tendon pain, localized tenderness and that is detrimental to an athletes performance. in the initial phase of the Jumper's knee injury the tendons with the knee are usually inflamed. If Jumper's knee becomes a chronic injury, which usually occurs as age increases, the tendons show an increasing degree of degeneration and little to no inflation present. As the etiology and pathology of Jumper's knee is not known the treatment varies and is largely based on a trial and error basis.

Jumpers knee is said to occur after frequent actions involving quick accelerations and declarations, eccentric activities and quick cutting actions. As spiking involves jumping, in which a quick acceleration occurs when jumping and quick deceleration when landing, this action is a possible cause of Jumper's knee. Also blocking is a possible cause of Jumper's knee because it to involves jumping and landing quickly. However, Jumper's knee is less common among athletes who compete in beach volleyball rather than those who play indoor volleyball. This is because beach volleyball is played on sand which reduces the impact of landing on the knee.

Patellar Tendinitis

Patellar tendinitis (patellar tendinopathy, also known as jumper's knee), is a relatively common cause of pain in the inferior patellar region in athletes. It is common with frequent jumping and studies have shown it may be associated with stiff ankle movement and ankle sprains.

Presentation

Jumper's knee (patellar tendinopathy, patellar tendinosis, patellar tendinitis) commonly occurs in athletes who are involved in jumping sports such as basketball and volleyball. Patients report anterior knee pain, often with an aching quality. The symptom onset is insidious. Rarely is a discrete injury described. Usually, involvement is infrapatellar at or near the infrapatellar pole, but it may also be suprapatellar.

Depending on the duration of symptoms, jumper's knee can be classified into 1 of 4 stages, as follows:

Stage 1 – Pain only after activity, without functional impairment

Stage 2 – Pain during and after activity, although the patient is still able to perform satisfactorily in his or her sport

Stage 3 – Prolonged pain during and after activity, with increasing difficulty in performing at a satisfactory level

Stage 4 – Complete tendon tear requiring surgical repair

It begins as inflammation in the patellar tendon where it attaches to the patella and may progress by tearing or degenerating the tendon. Patients present with an ache over the patella tendon. Most patients are between 10 and 16 years old. Magnetic resonance imaging can reveal edema (increased T2 signal intensity) in the proximal aspect of the patellar tendon.

Causes

It is an overuse injury from repetitive overloading of the extensor mechanism of the knee. The microtears exceed the body's healing mechanism unless the activity is stopped.

Among the risk factors for patellar tendonitis are low ankle dorsiflexion, weak gluteal muscles, and muscle tightness, particularly in the calves, quadriceps muscle, and hamstrings.

The injury occurs to athletes in many sports.

Treatment

Early stages may be treated conservatively using the R.I.C.E methods.

1. Rest
2. Ice
3. Compression
4. Elevation

Exercises involving eccentric muscle contractions of the quadriceps on a decline board are strongly supported by extant literature. A physical therapist may also recommend specific exercises and stretches to strengthen the muscles and tendons.

Should this fail, autologous blood injection, or platelet-rich plasma injection may be performed and is typically successful though not as successful as high volume saline injection (Crisp *et al.*). Uncommonly it may require surgery to remove myxoid degeneration in the tendon. This is reserved for patients with debilitating pain for 6–12 months despite conservative measures. Novel treatment modalities targeting the abnormal blood vessel growth which occurs in the condition are currently being investigated.

Tennis Injuries

Muscle strain is one of the most common injuries in tennis. When an isolated large-energy appears during the muscle contraction and at the same time body weight apply huge amount of pressure to the lengthened muscle which can result in the occurrence of muscle strain. Inflammation and bleeding are triggered when muscle strain occur which resulted in redness, pain and swelling. Overuse is also common in tennis players from all level. Muscle, cartilage, nerves, bursae, ligaments and tendons may be damaged from overuse. The repetitive use of a particular muscle without time for repair and recover in the most common case among the injury.

Types of Injuries

Lateral Epicondylitis

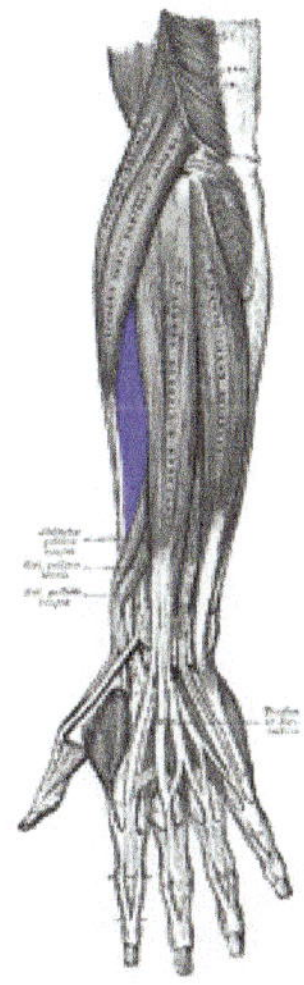

Coloured in purple: the Extensor Carpi Radialis Brevis muscle

Lateral epicondylitis is an overuse injury that frequently occur in tennis. It is also known as tennis elbow. This injury categorise as tendon injury where it occur in the forearm muscle called the extensor carpic radialis brevis (ECRB). The injury is regularly developed in the recreational players. Experienced players are less likely to develop lateral epicondylitis than the inexperienced players due to poorer technique. Tennis elbow or lateral epicondylalgia is a common injury that occurs in 40-50% of tennis players. It is more prominent at the lower levels of play and usually comes from any incorrect use of the wrist or grip on the forehand or one-handed backhand strokes. Players at higher levels often have more relaxed grips and have a larger racquet extension out to the ball after they make contact, where professionals have less emphasis on the arm and more on the use of every part of the body in order exert the natural power behind the ball, lower level players don't get the training to discover how to use their whole body for a tennis stroke and are often reduced to using their arms in order to exert all of the power therefore putting heavy strain on the arm. Holding the grip tightly will put more tension on the arm therefore when going for a swing the muscles will be absorbing all of the shock from the initial contact of the ball. Symptoms of tennis elbow include the slow pain which occurs around the elbow. Simple tasks such as shaking hands or moving the wrist with force, like lifting weights or doing push ups, will worsen the pain. Tennis Elbow has actually shown that inflammatory tendons are only part of the early stages or acute stages with a treatment of anti-inflammatory or steroids being appropriate uses for this symptom. Most players respond well to simple rest, but other means of treatment include physical therapy, strength training, and electrical stimulation. Some players make alterations to their racquet such as increasing grip size which will ultimately prevent any unwanted movement of the wrist when extending out and finishing the tennis stroke.

Shoulder

Shoulder injury is other common types of injury in tennis. Shoulder injury caused by the repetitive use of shoulder when serving and striking the ball. The injury also relevance to rotator cuffs pathology, toscapular dyskinesis or glenohumeral internal rotation deficit which leads to internal impingement and/or labral pathology. There is 24% of the high-level tennis players aged 12–19 suffered from shoulder pain and rise up to 50% for middle-aged players.

Back

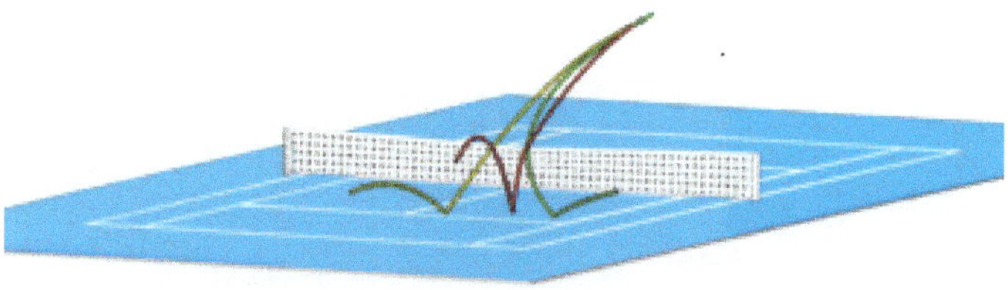

There are 3 different type of tennis serves. Yellow represent: Flat serve Red represent: Topspin serve Green represent: Slice serve

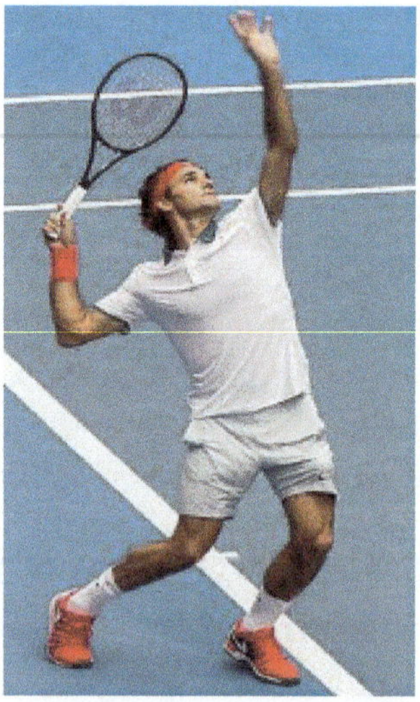

Roger Federer at Australian Open in 2014. Throughout his career back injury always been the problem for him.

It is common for tennis players in all level of play have experienced back injury throughout their career. In fact, more than 85% of the active athletes clarified that they have experienced back pain. According to 148 professional tennis player in one particular study, back pain forcing 39% of players to withdraw from the tournament. Furthermore, 29% of the player said they experienced chronic back pain. Lower back pain is the most common injury amongst tennis players with instances of postural abnormalities and general overuse which may occur during the back rotation and extension of the serve. In order to relieve pain in the lower back people are often told to rest it, but not for more than two days because of its potential damage to the bones, connecting tissue, and cardiovascular system. Once the back pain has dispersed stretching is recommended in order to prevent the stiffness from the initial pain, with examples being the squatting position or spinal extensions. In order to prevent future lower back injuries strength training to the abdominal muscles is necessary because with a stronger abdomen it will protect the back from excessive intervertebral disk strain. The straight crunch, the Oblique crunch, and balance exercises with the gym ball are some of the workouts for abdominal strengthening, but the exercises should be done with caution because if done incorrectly the strain on the back will be amplified. After the injury is dealt with, players of any level return to the court, the higher level players will often go through a thorough stretching period before any matches so they can assure that they won't hurt their back or any other part of their body.

Blister

Blister can be described as a patch that appears on the skin filled with a clear fluid and sometimes filled with blood. During physical activities, the continuous force of friction, cutting, squeezing and scratching which cause the separation of the epidermal cell layer, as a result the blister is formed. Blister (foot) occurs frequently among marathon runners, walk racers, backpackers and in hiking. In tennis, blister development site often occur on the hand or around the fingers because often time the skin is consistently rubbing against the tennis racquet.

Health Issues in Athletics

Health issues of athletics concern the health and well-being of athletes who participate in an organized sport. If athletes are physically and mentally underdeveloped, they are susceptible to mental or physical problems. Athletes trying to improve their performance in sports can harm themselves by overtraining, adopting eating habits that damage them physically or psychologically, and using steroids or supplements.

Female Athlete Triad

The Female Athlete Triad is a condition among women that consists of three related health irregularities: disordered eating habits, irregular menstruation, and premature bone loss or osteoporosis. The term was coined in the early 1990s when researchers from the National Institutes of Health noticed unusual health patterns among female athletes. These researchers observed increases in eating habit disorders in young female athletes. Exercising intensely while getting inadequate nutrition can lead to amenorrhea - or irregular menstrual cycles - which in turn can lead to osteoporosis.

Competitive Thinness

Female athletes tend to compare themselves to their competitors, which is another factor for athletes to develop female athlete triad. Competitive thinness is a term used when athletes compare themselves to their rivals who are performing better than them. When athletes begin to compare themselves to their competitors and notice the athletes who are performing better than them are thinner, it can lead to a weight loss mentality. Another risk factor to competitive thinness is related to revealing uniforms. For aesthetic sports, these uniforms are normally very tight, which shows off the athletes' body. These uniforms can cause athletes to develop unhealthy body comparisons.

Over-training

A female athlete who feels pressured to maintain a certain physique or body weight may exercise excessively and develop eating disorders to restrict calorie intake. Over-exercising increases the need for rest; her overall energy declines, causing her total body fat and estrogen levels to drop - a condition known as amenorrhea. Both male and female athletes may feel the pressure to over-train excessively in order to achieve a certain body image. The human body has a tremendous capacity to adapt to physical stress. "Stress" does not mean only physical damage. It can also refer to activity beneficial to bones, muscles, tendons, and ligaments, making them stronger and more functional. This is also known as "remodeling," and involves both the breakdown and buildup of tissue. However, if breakdown occurs more rapidly than buildup, an overuse injury can result. Nearly half of all injuries encountered in pediatric sports medicine are due to overuse. An overuse injury is traumatic damage to a bone, muscle, or tendon that is subjected to repetitive stress without time to heal naturally, as a result of long and/or high-intensity workouts. Many young athletes participate in sports year-round or on multiple teams at once. Another factor could be parental pressure to compete and succeed. Other risk factors include sleep deprivation, general physical and cognitive immaturity, dietary imbalance and inadequate physical fitness. Among young athletes, a common form of overuse injury is stress fractures, which include injuries of the:

- femoral neck/pubis
- femoral shaft
- tibia
- fibula

- metatarsals
- calcaneus
- cuboid

'Over-training Syndrome' is a term that has been used to describe athletes who, while training for competition, train beyond the body's ability to recover naturally. Common warning signs include tiredness, soreness, drop in performance, headaches, and loss of enthusiasm. Without adequate rest and recovery, training regimens can backfire, eventually harming an athlete's performance. Over-training can also be associated with eating disorders; athletes can turn to excessive exercise in order to lose weight. In cases where athletes are over-training, the most effective treatment is rest and proper nutrition.

Supplements/Steroids

Anabolic steroids are artificially produced hormones called androgens, which are essentially male-type sex hormones in the body. The most powerful of the androgens is testosterone. Another group of steroids are steroidal supplements, a weaker form of androgens. Steroids and supplements are controversial when used for sports because of the health risks associated with them. Some serious and long-term effects on the body are hair loss, dizziness, mood swings, delusions, paranoia, high blood pressure, and increased risk of heart disease, stroke, and even cancer. More recent studies also suggest that steroid users have an increased risk of depression and alcohol use later in life. Doctors call this the 'snowball effect' of steroid-related health problems. Injury patterns suggest that joint ligaments are not able to adapt to steroid-enhanced muscles, leading to injury.

Heat Illness

Heat illness and dehydration are typically brought on by high temperatures and high humidity. These conditions carry increased risk for young athletes, particularly at the beginning of a season, when they are less fit. Other factors that increase vulnerability include: heat-retaining clothing, recent illness, previous experience with heat illness, chronic conditions, and sleep deprivation. Additional precautions should be taken if a child is taking supplements or using cold medication.

Heat illnesses are among the primary causes of sports-related death or disability. They require immediate medical attention. Symptoms to watch for are as follows:

- dry or sticky mouth
- headache
- dizziness

- cramps
- unusual fatigue
- confusion
- loss of consciousness

Injury

Sports injuries are often the result of overuse or trauma to a part of the body. An issue unique to youth athletics is that the participants' bones are still growing, making them especially at risk for injury. Around 8,000 children are rushed to the emergency room daily because of sports injuries. High school athletes suffer approximately 715,000 injuries annually. In American football, for instance, five times as many catastrophic injuries happen in high school as in college-level competition. Injuries include heat illness and dehydration, concussions, and trauma-related deaths. Heat illnesses are a rising concern in youth athletics. These illnesses include heat syncope, muscle cramps, heat exhaustion, heat stroke and exertional hyponatremia. Each year, high school athletes sustain 300,000 head injuries, of which 90% are concussions. By the start of high school, 53% of athletes will have already suffered a concussion, but fewer than 50% of them say anything because they are concerned they will be removed from play. Ice hockey, soccer, lacrosse, wrestling and basketball have a high risk of concussion, with football carrying the most risk. A history of concussion in a football player can contribute to sports-related sudden death.

Prevention

To prevent an injury, proper warm-up is extremely important, because it lets athletes increase their heart rates. Proper warm-up also increases muscle temperature. Warm muscles are less susceptible to injuries because they can contract more forcefully and relax more quickly. As a result, both speed and strength can be enhanced. Also, the probability of over-stretching a muscle and causing injury is much lower. Warm-ups also increase body and blood temperature, which allows more oxygen to reach the muscles, improves muscle elasticity, and reduces the risk of strains and pulls. Other forms of prevention include strengthening muscles, increasing flexibility, taking breaks, weight training, and playing safe. Mental preparation is also important before practice or games. Clearing the mind and visualizing skills and strategy can relax the athlete's muscles and build concentration.

Sports-related Death

Sometimes sports injuries can be so severe that they lead to death. In 2010 48 youths died from sports injuries. The leading causes of death in youth sports are sudden cardiac arrest, concussion, heat illness and external sickling. Cardiac-related deaths are usually due to an undiagnosed cardiovascular disorder. Trauma to the head, neck and spine can also be lethal. Among young American athletes, more than half of trauma-related deaths take place among football players, with track and field, lacrosse, baseball, boxing, and soccer also having relatively high fatality rates.

Health Issues in Youth Sports

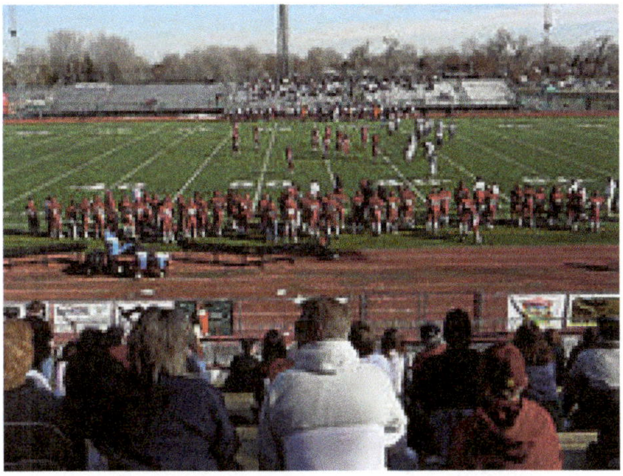

Rocky Mountain High School, football field

The health issues of youth sports are concerns regarding the health and wellbeing of young people between the ages of 6 and 18 who participate in an organized sport. Given that these athletes are physically and mentally underdeveloped, they are particularly susceptible to heat illness, eating disorders and injury; sufficiently severe conditions can result in death.

Heat Illness and Dehydration

Heat illnesses are a recent concern in youth athletics. They include heat syncope, muscle cramps, heat exhaustion, heat stroke and exertional hyponatremia. Heat illness and dehydration are typically brought on by conditions of high temperatures and high humidity. These conditions carry increased risk for young athletes, particularly if at the beginning of a season when they are less fit. Other factors which increase vulnerability include: heat-retaining clothing, recent illness, previous experience with heat illness, chronic conditions, or sleep deprivation. Additional precaution is to be taken if the child is taking supplements or using cold medication.

Heat illnesses are among the primary causes of sports-related death or disability, and as such they require immediate medical attention. Symptoms to watch for are as follows:

- dry or sticky mouth
- headache

- dizziness
- cramps
- unusual fatigue
- confusion
- loss of consciousness

Eating Disorders

Eating disorders are generally not a primary concern amongst youth athletes, however they are unusually prevalent in wrestling and aesthetic sports such as gymnastics. These place heavy emphasis upon weight and body image as ingredients for success in competition. In order to compete, 81% of wrestlers will deliberately lose weight. This involves shedding 3% to 20% of their body weight — most of which being dropped within a short period of time. For rhythmic gymnasts, "success is strongly influenced by visual appeal and body aesthetics. Rhythmic gymnasts are often required to meet certain weight targets to attain and maintain a thin shape." The pressure to please is intense, and correspondingly, 42% of female aesthetic athletes have been diagnosed with eating disorders.

Youth athletes employ a variety of methods to lose weight, including dehydration, fasting, diet pills, laxatives, vomiting, and the use of rubber exercise suits. These practices result in "decreased plasma and blood volume, reduced cardiac outputs, impaired thermoregulatory responses, decreased renal blood flow, and an increase in the amount of electrolytes lost from the body."

Long-term Effects

It has been postulated that wrestlers may suffer impaired growth and development due to their fluctuating body weight. However, a study examining high school wrestler growth patterns concluded that participation does not stunt growth. In relation to eating disorders, young female gymnasts may suffer from delayed menarche, menstrual irregularities, low body fat, and delayed maturity. Of these athletes, 11% are at risk for a mental disorder, while 40% risk delayed physical maturation.

Injuries

An issue unique to youth athletics is that the participants' bones are still growing, placing them at highest risk for injury. Around 8,000 children are rushed to the emergency room daily because of sports injuries. High school athletes suffer approximately 715,000 injuries annually. Regarding American football, there are five times more catastrophic injuries in high school than compared to college-level competition.

Overuse Injuries

Nearly half of all injuries in pediatric sports medicine are due to overuse. Such injuries can be attributed to inappropriate workout intensity and overlong athletic seasons. Other risk factors include sleep deprivation, general physical and cognitive immaturity, dietary imbalance and inadequate physical fitness. Among young athletes, common overuse injuries are stress fractures, which include injury of the:

- femoral neck/pubis
- femoral shaft
- tibia
- fibula
- metatarsals
- calcaneus
- cuboid

Concussions

Per year, high school athletes sustain 300,000 head injuries, 90% of which being concussions. Though by the beginning of high school, 53% of athletes will have already suffered a concussion. Less than 50% of them say something about it in order to stay in the game. If an athlete returns to competition before being completely healed, they are more susceptible to suffer another concussion. A repeat concussion can have a much slower recovery rate and be accompanied by increased symptoms and long-term effects. The severity of complications from concussion can include brain swelling, blood clots and brain damage. Ice hockey, soccer, wrestling and basketball carry a high risk for concussion, with football at the top.). Concussion causing situations that involve leading with the head, hitting head to head and striking a defenseless athlete have become subject to penalty in order to discourage players and coaches from this type of play. These rule changes have resulted in technique changes at the youngest levels of sports, and youth athletes are now being trained in methods avoiding illegal contact. Youth sport organizations have also made equipment changes to better protect players. A widespread myth is that helmets protect athletes from concussions; they are actually worn to prevent skull fractures. Facts like this have prompted trainings on proper equipment use and not relying on helmets as an implement of contact. A history of concussion in football players can contribute to sports-related sudden death.

Sports-related Death

Sometimes sports injuries can be so severe as to result in actual death. Over the past year, 48 youths died from sports injuries. The leading causes of death in youth sports are sudden cardiac arrest, concussion, heat illness and external sickling. Cardiac-related deaths are usually due to an undiagnosed cardiovascular disorder. Trauma to the head, neck and spine can also be lethal. Among young American athletes, more than half of trauma-related deaths are to football players, with track and field, baseball, boxing and soccer also having relatively high fatality rates.

Female Athlete Triad

Female athlete triad is a syndrome in which eating disorders (or *low energy availability*), amenorrhoea/*oligomenorrhoea*, and *decreased bone mineral density* (osteoporosis and osteopenia) are present. Also known simply as the Triad, this condition is seen in females participating in sports that emphasize leanness or low body weight. The triad is a serious illness with lifelong health consequences and can potentially be fatal.

Classification

The female athlete triad is a syndrome of three interrelated conditions. Thus, if an athlete is suffering from one element of the Triad, it is likely that she is suffering from the other two components of the triad as well. With the increase in female participation in sports, much of it attributable to Title IX legislation in the United States, the incidence of a triad of disorders particular to women — the female athlete triad—has also increased. Due to this increasing prevalence, the female athlete triad and its relationship with athletics was identified in the 1980s as the symptoms, risk factors, causes and treatments were studied in depth and their relatedness evaluated. The condition is most common in cross country running, gymnastics, and figure skating. Many of those who suffer from the triad are involved in some sort of athletics, in order to promote weight loss and leanness. The competitive sports that promote this physical leanness may result in disordered eating, and be responsible for the origin of the Female Athlete Triad. For some women, not balancing the needs of their bodies and their sports can have major consequences. In addition, for some competitive female athletes, problems such as low self-esteem, a tendency toward perfectionism, and family stress place them at risk for disordered eating.

Signs and Symptoms

Clinical symptoms of the Triad may include disordered eating, fatigue, hair loss, cold hands and feet, dry skin, noticeable weight loss, increased healing time from injuries (e.g., lingering bruises), increased incidence of bone fracture and cessation of menses. Affected females may also struggle with low self-esteem and depression.

Upon physical examination, a physician may also note the following symptoms: elevated carotene in the blood, anemia, orthostatic hypotension, electrolyte irregularities, hypoestrogenism, vaginal atrophy, and bradycardia.

An athlete may show signs of restrictive eating, but not meet the clinical criteria for an eating disorder. She may also display subtle menstrual disturbances, such as a change in menstrual cycle length, anovulation, or luteal phase defects, but not yet have developed complete amenorrhea. Likewise, an athlete's bone density may decrease, but may not yet have dropped below her age-matched normal range. These signs can be considered "occult," as no one symptom may be severe enough to seek medical attention, leaving the Triad to go unnoticed or untreated.

Eating Disorder

Energy availability is defined as energy intake minus energy expended. Energy is taken in through food consumption. Our bodies expend energy through normal functioning as well as through exercise. In the case of female athlete triad, low energy availability may be due to eating disorders, but not necessarily so. Athletes may experience low energy availability by exercising more without a concomitant change in eating habits, or they may increase their energy expenditure while also eating less. Disordered eating is defined among this situation due to the low caloric intake or low energy availability.

While most athletes do not meet the clinical criteria to be diagnosed with an eating disorder such as anorexia nervosa or bulimia nervosa, many will exhibit disordered eating habits such as fasting, as well as avoiding certain types of food the athlete thinks are "bad" (such as foods containing fat). More severe examples of disordered eating habits may include binge-eating; purging; and the use of diet-pills, laxatives, diuretics, and enemas.

By restricting their diet, the athlete may worsen their problem of low energy availability. Having low dietary energy from excessive exercise and/or dietary restrictions leaves too little energy for the body to carry out normal functions such as maintaining a regular menstrual cycle or healthy bone density.

Amenorrhea

Amenorrhea, defined as the cessation of a woman's menstrual cycle for more than three months, is the second disorder in the Triad. Weight fluctuations from dietary restrictions and/or excessive exercise affect the hypothalamus's output of gonadotropic hormones. Gonadotropic hormones "stimulate growth of the gonads and the secretion of sex hormones." (e.g. gonadotropin-releasing hormone, lutenizing hormone and follicle stimulating hormone.) These gonadotropic hormones play a role in stimulating estrogen release from the ovaries. Without estrogen release, the menstrual cycle is disrupted. Exercising intensely and not eating enough calories can lead to decreases in estrogen, the hormone that helps to regulate the menstrual cycle. As a result, a female's periods may become irregular or stop altogether.

There are two types of amenorrhea. A woman who has been having her period and then stops menstruating for ninety days or more is said to have secondary amenorrhea. Primary amenorrhea is characterized by delayed menarche (the onset of menses during puberty). Delayed menarche may be associated with delay of the development of secondary sexual characteristics.

Osteoporosis

Osteoporosis is defined by the National Institutes of Health as "a skeletal disorder characterized by compromised bone strength predisposing a person to an increased risk of fracture." Low estrogen levels and poor nutrition, especially low calcium intake, can lead to osteoporosis, the third aspect of the triad. This condition can ruin a female athlete's career because it may lead to stress fractures and other injuries.

Patients with female athlete triad get osteoporosis due to hypoestrogenemia, or low estrogen levels. With estrogen deficiency, the osteoclasts live longer and are therefore able to resorb more bone. In response to the increased bone resorption, there is increased bone formation and a high-turnover state develops which leads to bone loss and perforation of the trabecular plates. As osteoclasts break down bone, patients see a loss of bone mineral density. Low bone mineral density renders bones more brittle and hence susceptible to fracture. Because athletes are active and their bones must endure mechanical stress, the likelihood of experiencing bone fracture is particularly high.

Additionally, because those suffering with female athlete triad are also restricting their diet, they may also not be consuming sufficient amounts vitamins and minerals which contribute to bone density; not getting enough calcium or vitamin D further exacerbates the problem of weak bones.

Bone mass is now thought to peak between the ages of 18-25. Thus, behaviors which result in low bone density in youth could be detrimental to an athlete's bone health throughout her lifetime.

Causes

Gymnastics, figure skating, ballet, diving, swimming, and long distance running are examples of sports which emphasize low body weight. The Triad is seen more often in aesthetic sports such as these versus ball game sports. Women taking part in these sports may be at an increased risk for developing female athlete triad.

Athletes at greatest risk for low energy availability are those who restrict dietary energy intake, who exercise for prolonged periods, who are vegetarian, and who limit the types of food they will eat. Many factors appear to contribute to disordered eating behaviors and clinical eating disorders. Dieting is a common entry point and interest has focused on the contribution of environmental and social factors, psychological predisposition, low self-esteem, family dysfunction, abuse, biological factors, and genetics. Additional factors for athletes include early start of sport-specific training and dieting, injury, and a sudden increase in training volume. Surveys show more negative eating attitude scores in athletic disciplines favoring leanness. Disordered eating behaviors are risk factors for eating disorders.

Treatment

The underlying cause of the female athlete triad is an imbalance between energy taken into the body (through nutrition) and energy used by the body (through exercise). The treatment includes correcting this imbalance by either increasing calories in a diet or by decreasing calories burned by exercise for 12 months or longer. Persons with female athlete triad should get treatment from a multi-disciplinary team that includes a physician, dietitian, and mental health counselor, and seek support from family, friends, and their coach.

Because a symptom of the female athlete triad is menstrual dysfunction, some physicians may recommend oral contraceptives because those pills will regulate the menstrual cycle. However, the underlying cause of the menstrual disorder is an energy imbalance, and using pills to regulate the menstrual cycle without changes in diet and behavior is likely to mask the food deficiency and delay appropriate treatment. A woman taking contraceptives to treat menstrual dysfunction without correcting this energy imbalance will continue to lose bone density.

Less Exercise

Continued participation in training and competition depends on the physical and mental health of the athlete. Athletes who weigh less than 80 percent of their ideal body weight may not be able to safely participate.

Persons with female athlete triad are often asked by health care providers to reduce the amount of time they spend exercising by 10-12 percent.

Eating More

Low energy availability with or without eating disorders, functional hypothalamic amenorrhea, and osteoporosis, alone or in combination, pose significant health risks to physically active girls and women. Prevention, recognition, and treatment of these clinical conditions should be a priority of those who work with female athletes to ensure that they maximize the benefits of regular exercise.

Patients are recommended to work with a dietician who can monitor their nutritional status and help the patient work towards a healthy goal weight. Patients should also meet with a psychiatrist or psychologist to address the psychological aspects of the triad. Therefore, it is important that trainers and coaches are made aware of the athlete's condition and be part of her recovery.

Medicine

Patients are also sometimes treated pharmacologically. To both induce menses and improve bone density, doctors may prescribe cyclic estrogen or progesterone as is used to treat post-menopausal women. Patients may also be put on oral contraceptives to stimulate regular periods. In addition to hormone therapy, nutrition supplements may be recommended. Doctors may prescribe calcium supplements. Vitamin D supplements may be also used because this vitamin aids in calcium absorption. Bisphosphonates and calcitonin, used to treat adults with osteoporosis, may be prescribed, although their effectiveness in adolescents has not yet been established. Finally, if indicated by a psychiatric examination, the affected athlete may be prescribed anti-depressants and in some cases benzodiazepines to help in alleviating severe distress at mealtimes.

Prognosis

Sustained low energy availability, with or without disordered eating, can impair health. Psychological problems associated with eating disorders include low self-esteem, depression, and anxiety disorders. Medical complications involve the cardiovascular, endocrine, reproductive, skeletal, gastrointestinal, renal, and central nervous systems. The prognosis for anorexia nervosa is grave with a six-fold increase in standard mortality rates compared to the general population. In one study, 5.4% of athletes with eating disorders reported suicide attempts. Although 83% of anorexia nervosa patients partially recover, the rate of sustained recovery of weight, menstrual function and eating behavior is only 33%.

Amenorrheic women can be infertile, due to the absence of ovarian follicular development, ovulation, and luteal function. Consequences of hypoestrogenism seen in amenorrheic athletes include impaired endothelium-dependent arterial vasodilation, which reduces the perfusion of working muscle, impaired skeletal muscle oxidative metabolism, elevated low-density lipoprotein cholesterol levels, and vaginal dryness.

Due to low bone mineral density that declines as the number of missed menstrual cycles accumulates, and the loss of BMD may not be fully reversible. Stress fractures occur more commonly in physically active women with menstrual irregularities and/or low BMD with a relative risk for stress fracture two to four times greater in amenorrheic than eumenorrheic athletes. Fractures also occur in the setting of nutritional deficits and low BMD.

Society and Culture

The American Academy of Pediatrics and the AAFP contend that exercise is important and should be promoted in girls for health and enjoyment, however pediatricians should be wary of health problems that may occur in female athlete. The health related issues concerning this topic are grave and can lead to numerous health issues as previously demonstrated. The treatment plan will depend on the severity of the disorder, however some form of treatment has been shown as helpful to produce successful progress towards a better health condition. Clearly, many health problems arise due to disordered eating.

Coaches are discouraged from active participation in the treatment of eating disorders. In addition to conflicts of interest, coaches may be perceived to pressure athletes and potentially perpetuate components of the Female Athlete Triad. For example, in maintaining a place on the team or continued scholarship support, a female athlete may feel compelled to overtrain or restrict eating.

Moving Forward

Coaches, athletic trainers, and healthcare providers should also be educated about the female athlete triad to detect and recognize its components before athletes reach the pathologic end of the spectrum. Awareness levels among athletes, coaches, and healthcare professionals should be assessed to determine where education is needed most. A patient may present with any of the components of the triad; therefore, an awareness of these components among all involved in the care of female athletes is prudent. Athletes should also be taught proper nutrition for athletic performance by their coaches and health providers, because a specific breakdown of macronutrients combined with healthy dietary choices will help these athletes perform the best they possibly can, instead of forcing them to only care about their physique.

The female triad may also present in para-athletes.

References

- Ferguson, R. J., Mcmaster, J. H., & Stanitski, C. L. (1974). "Low back pain in college football linemen.". The American Journal of Sports Medicine. 2 (2): 63–69. doi:10.1177/036354657400200201. CS1 maint: Multiple names: authors list (link)
- Levangie, P. K., & Norkin, C. C. (2011). Joint structure and function: A comprehensive analysis (5th ed.). Philadelphia: F.A. Davis Co. ISBN 9780803623620. CS1 maint: Multiple names: authors list (link)
- Rivara, G R (2014). "Sports-Related Concussions in Youth: Improving the Science, Changing the Culture". Institute of Medicine; National Research Council. Retrieved 12 November 2014
- Öztürk, Selcen. "What is the economic burden of sports injuries?" (PDF). Joint Diseases and Related Surgery. 24 (2): 108–111. doi:10.5606/ehc.2013.24
- Eriksson, K., Nemeth, G., & Eriksson, E. (1996). "Low back pain in elite cross-country skiers.". Scandinavian journal of medicine & science in sports. 1 (6): 31–35. doi:10.1111/j.1600-0838.1996.tb00067.x. CS1 maint: Multiple names: authors list (link)
- Smith, Julian; Joe J. Tjandra; Gordon J. A. Clunie; Kaye, Andrew H. (2006). Textbook of Surgery. Wiley-Blackwell. p. 446. ISBN 1-4051-2627-2
- Gibson, Owen (November 4, 2013). "Concussion Rules under Spotlight in Wake of Hugo Lloris Row". The Guardian. Retrieved March 21, 2016

- Cantu RC (2007). "Chronic traumatic encephalopathy in the National Football League". Neurosurgery. 61 (2): 223–5. PMID 17762733. doi:10.1227/01.NEU.0000255514.73967.90
- Mendonça, Luciana (2011). "Correlation between isokinetic profile and shoulder injuries in male volleyball athletes". British journal of sports medicine. 45: 343. doi:10.1136/bjsm.2011.084038.93
- Bailes, Julian (2001). Neurological Sports Medicine: A Guide for Physicians and Athletic Trainers. Rolling Meadows, Illinois: Thieme. ISBN 1879284758
- "Cheerleading is leading cause of catastrophic injury in young women". University of Michigan Health System. 3 August 2009. Retrieved 2013-04-15
- Tysvaer AT (September 1992). "Head and neck injuries in soccer. Impact of minor trauma". Sports Med. 14 (3): 200–13. PMID 1439395. doi:10.2165/00007256-199214030-00006
- Bahr, Roald (1994). "Incidence and mechanisms of acute ankle inversion injuries in volleyball: A retrospective cohort study". The American Journal of Sports Medicine
- Terry R. Yochum; Lindsay J. Rowe (2004). Essentials of Skeletal Radiology (3rd ed.). Baltimore, MD: Lippincott Williams & Wilkins. ISBN 0781739462
- Owens, Brett D; Moriatis Wolf, Jennifer; Murphy, Kevin P (2009-11-03). "Lateral Epicondylitis: Workup". eMedicine Orthopedic Surgery. Retrieved 2010-04-19
- Barber, F. Alan; Sutker, Allan N. (August 1992). "Iliotibial Band Syndrome". Sports Medicine. 14 (2): 144–148. doi:10.2165/00007256-199214020-00005
- Bowen AP (2003). "Second impact syndrome: A rare, catastrophic, preventable complication of concussion in young athletes". Journal of Emergency Nursing. 29 (3): 287–289. PMID 12776088. doi:10.1067/men.2003.90
- Caine, Dennis J.; Maffulli, Nicola, eds. (2005). Epidemiology of Pediatric Sports Injuries. Medicine and Sport Science. 48. Karger Publishers. ISBN 9783805578684
- "Pitcher's Elbow - Stanford Sports Medicine - Stanford Medical Outpatient Center". Stanford University Medical Center. Retrieved 9 September 2009
- Reid, D.C.; Saboe, L. (June 1989). "Spine Fractures in Winter Sports". Sports Medicine. Adis International. 7 (6): 393–399. ISSN 0112-1642. PMID 2662325. doi:10.2165/00007256-198907060-00004
- Terrell TR (2004). "Concussion in athletes" (PDF). Southern Medical Journal. 97 (9): 837–842. PMID 15455966. doi:10.1097/01.SMJ.0000140091.58338.1E
- McKeag, Douglas; Moeller, James L. (2007-01-01). ACSM's Primary Care Sports Medicine. Lippincott Williams & Wilkins. ISBN 9780781770286
- J. Gould, Douglas. "The neuroanatomical relationship of Dementia Pugilistica and Alzheimer's Disease" (PDF). Neuroanatomy. Retrieved 1 April 2013

4

Understanding Sports Medicine

The branch of medicine which deals with injuries caused by physical exercise is known as sports medicine. The common types of injuries that occur because of sports are muscle cramps, ACL tears, shin splints, concussion, muscle strains and ACL sprains. This chapter discusses sports medicince in a critical manner providing key analysis to the subject matter.

Sports Medicine

Sports medicine, also known as sport and exercise medicine (SEM), is a branch of medicine that deals with physical fitness and the treatment and prevention of injuries related to sports and exercise. Although most sports teams have employed team physicians for many years, it is only since the late 20th century that sports medicine has emerged as a distinct field of health care.

Scope

Sport and exercise medicine doctors are specialist physicians who have completed medical school, appropriate residency training and then specialize further in sports medicine or 'sports and exercise medicine' (the preferred term). Specialization in sports medicine may be a doctor's first specialty (as in Australia, Netherlands, Norway, Italy). It may also be a sub-specialty or second specialisation following a specialisation such as physiatry or orthopedic surgery. The various approaches reflect the medical culture in different countries.

Specializing in the treatment of athletes and other physically active individuals, sports and exercise medicine physicians have extensive education in musculoskeletal medicine. SEM doctors treat injuries such as muscle, ligament, tendon and bone problems, but may also treat chronic illnesses that can affect physical performance, such as asthma and diabetes. SEM doctors also advise on managing and preventing injuries.

Specialists in SEM diagnose and treat any medical conditions which regular exercisers or sports persons encounter. The majority of an SEM physician's time is therefore spent treating musculoskeletal injuries, however other conditions include sports cardiology issues, unexplained underperformance syndrome, exercise-induced asthma, screening for cardiac abnormalities and diabetes in sports. In addition team physicians working in elite sports often play a role in performance medicine, whereby an athletes' physiology is monitored, and aberrations corrected, in order to achieve peak physical performance.

SEM consultants also deliver clinical physical activity interventions, negating the burden of disease directly attributable to physical inactivity and the compelling evidence for the effectiveness of exercise in the primary, secondary and tertiary prevention of disease.

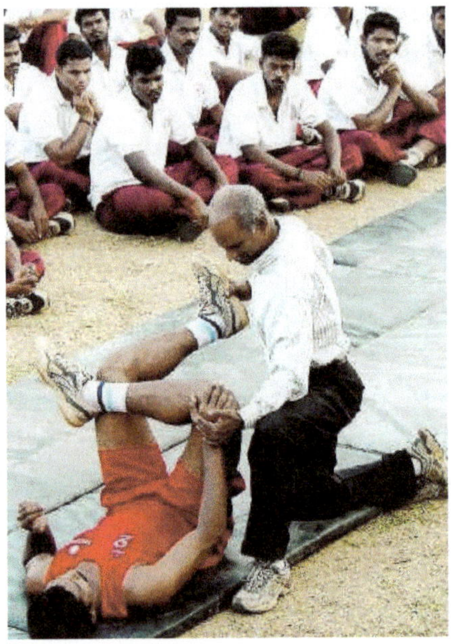

Exercise Medicine

The Foresight Report issued by the UK's Government Office for Science, 17 October 2007, highlighted the unsustainable health and economic costs of a nation that continues to be largely sedentary. It forecasts that the incremental costs of this inactivity will be $10 billion per year by 2050 and the wider costs to society and businesses $49.9billion. Physical inactivity inevitably leads to ill-health and it forecasts the cost of paying for this impact will be unsustainable in the future. No existing group of medical specialists is equipped with the skills and training to deal with this challenge.

Public Health

SEM physicians are frequently involved in promoting the therapeutic benefits of physical activity, exercise and sport for the individuals and communities. SEM Physicians in the UK spend a period of their training in public health, and advise public health physicians on matters relating to physical activity promotion. An example of published work includes the Royal College of Physicians publications.

Common Sports Injuries

Concussion – caused by severe head injury where the brain moves violently within the skull so that brain cells all fire at once, much like a seizure.

Muscle cramps – a sudden tight, intense pain caused by a muscle locked in spasm. Muscle cramps are also recognized as an involuntary and forcibly contracted muscle that does not relax.

ACL sprains – The anterior cruciate ligament (ACL) is a ligament involved in knee stabilization. An ACL rupture can occur when the foot is planted and the knee twists to change direction.

ACL tears – The anterior cruciate ligament; one of four major knee ligament necessary for comfortable knee movement, tears, causing major pain and causes the knee to "give out". The knee ACL can tear for a number of reasons.

Ankle sprain – The ligaments that hold the ankle bones in place can easily be overstretched.

Shin splints – The tissue that attaches the muscles of the lower leg to the shin bone may be pulling away from the bone, or it may be inflamed from overuse.

Muscle strains – tears in muscle that cause pain and or loss of function.

History

In recent years Western society has increasingly recognized the dangers of physical inactivity, and significant efforts have been made within the public health community to encourage the nation to become more physically active. To reflect this paradigm shift BASM has renamed itself BASEM (British Association of Sport and Exercise Medicine) and the speciality itself has rebranded from Sports Medicine to Sport & Exercise Medicine. Since 2007 several deaneries across the UK have established training programmes in SEM, and recurrent funding for 50 National Training Numbers (NTN's) is available.

Organizations

- American College of Sports Medicine (ACSM) Founded in 1954, the American College of Sports Medicine is the largest and most prominent sports medicine and exercise science organization in the world. ACSM has more than 45,000 International, National and Regional Chapter members.
- American Orthopaedic Society for Sports Medicine (AOSSM) The American Orthopaedic Society for Sports Medicine is a world leader in sports medicine education, research, communication, and fellowship. Founded in 1972,

AOSSM is an international organization of orthopaedic surgeons and other allied health professionals dedicated to sports medicine. Essentially every professional and collegiate team has a team physician who is a member of the AOSSM.

- American Medical Society for Sports Medicine (AMSSM) AMSSM is a multi-disciplinary organization of sports medicine physicians dedicated to education, research, advocacy and the care of athletes of all ages. The majority of AMSSM members are primary care physicians with fellowship training and added qualification in sports medicine who then combine their practice of sports medicine with their primary specialty. AMSSM includes members who specialize solely in non-surgical sports medicine and serve as team physicians at the youth level, NCAA, NFL, MLB, NBA, WNBA, MLS and NHL, as well as with Olympic teams. By nature of their training and experience, sports medicine physicians are ideally suited to provide comprehensive medical care for athletes, sports teams or active individuals who are simply looking to maintain a healthy lifestyle.
- National Athletic Trainers' Association (NATA) Founded in 1950, the mission of the National Athletic Trainers Association is to enhance the quality of health care provided by certified athletic trainers and to advance the athletic training profession.
- Canadian Athletic Therapists' Association (CATA) Founded in 1965. The Canadian Athletic Therapists Association (CATA) is an organization devoted to the comprehensive health care of an individual at any level of physical ability by Certified Athletic Therapists.
- American Medical Association (AMA) The American Medical Association recognized Athletic Training(AT) as an allied health profession in 1990.
- International Society of Arthroscopy, Knee Surgery and Sports Medicine (ISAKOS) The ISAKOS - International Society of Arthroscopy, Knee Surgery and Orthopaedic Sports Medicine is an international society with over 4,000 surgeons members, dedicated to advancing of education, research and patient care in arthroscopy, knee surgery and orthopaedic sports medicine around the world.
- International Association for Dance Medicine and Science (IADMS) The International Association for Dance Medicine & Science was formed in 1990 by an international group of dance medicine practitioners, dance educators, dance scientists, and dancers. Membership is drawn equally from the medical and dance professions, and has grown from an initial 48 members in 1991 to over 900 members at present worldwide, representing 35 countries.

Athletic Taping

Athletic taping is the process of applying tape directly to the skin in order to maintain a stable position of bones and muscles during athletic activity. It is a procedure that uses tape, attached to the skin, to physically keep in place muscles or bones at a certain position. This reduces pain and aids recovery. Taping is usually used to help recover from overuse and other injuries.

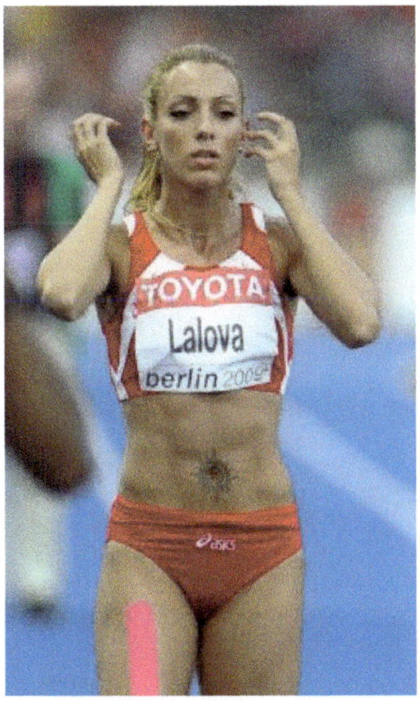

Taping on Ivet Lalova

The general goals of athletic taping are to restrict the motion of an injured joint, compress soft tissues to reduce swelling, support anatomical structures involved in the injury, serve as a splint or secure a splint, secure dressing or bandages, protect the injured joint from re-injury, and protect the injured part while the injured part is in the healing process.

Role of Taping

Taping has many roles such as to support the ligaments and capsules of unstable joints by limiting excessive or abnormal anatomical movement. Taping also enhances proprioceptive feedback from the limb or joint. Finally taping can support injuries at the muscle-tendon units by compressing and limiting movement and secure protective pads, dressings and splints.

Advantages

Injury Prevention: Athletic taping is recognized as one of the top preventative measures for reduction of injuries in collision sports. These injuries often occur as a result of extrinsic factors such as collision with other players or equipment. Athletic taping has also been shown to reduce the severity in injuries, as well as the occurrence of injury in most sports.

Injury Management: Tape is often applied to manage symptoms of chronic injuries such as medial tibial stress syndrome (or shin splints), patella-femoral syndrome, and turf-toe. Athletic tape can be applied to ease pain symptoms as well. Taping along the nerve tract of irritated or inflamed tissue can shorten the inflamed region and reduce pain.

Other post-injury benefits include: 1) stabilizing and supporting joints after injuries to the muscle or ligament; 2) assisting and allowing the athlete to return to activity after minor injuries; 3) preventing and reducing further harm to injured area; 4) maintaining proper biomechanics during activity; 5) preventing neuromuscular damage; and 6) reducing force on the area during activity.

Disadvantages

- Incorrect athletic taping may lead to blistering or future injuries.
- After activity and motion begins, the stiffness of the tape reduces.
- Physiological dependency on using tape
- Expensive, especially when it is needed frequently

Techniques

There are set regulations and rules that govern the athletic taping techniques used by trainers and health professionals. There are a few aspects of athletic taping that are standardized.

1. Skin preparation: Removal of hair, cleaning of skin, addressing of any lesions with necessary consultation, using adherents and lubricants, underpads, etc.
2. Functional position of the body to be taped: The athlete's position depends on the area getting taped.
3. Body mechanics of the trainer/taper: The athlete must be at a comfortable height in order to reduce fatigue over long periods of taping time.
4. Athletic tape application: Athletic tape must be adhered to a dry and clean area of the body at body temperature to bare skin or pre-wrap in order to prevent slippage and to maintain the effectiveness and rigidity of the wrap. The type and width of the athletic tape must be appropriate (able to strap the given body part suitable) for the area being taped. Areas subject to high friction should be reinforced with protective padding or under-wrap. Athletic tape should be

applied: film and wrinkle free; without impairment of circulation, nerves, or muscle movement; and without pressure on body prominences.

5. Removal: Removal of the athletic tape post athletic activity should be done with tape cutters (sometimes known as 'Sharks') or special tape scissors. The skin must be free of tape residue.

Applications

Upper Limbs and Chest (Thorax)

- Shoulder
  - Shoulder
  - Shoulder including the arm
- Thorax
- Upper limb
  - Elbow
  - Wrist
  - Wrist only
  - Wrist including thumb
  - Fingers
- Thumb
- Finger

Inferior Limbs

- Thigh
- Knee
- Achilles' heel
  - Preventive
  - Alleviating
- Ankle
- Foot
- Toes
  - Hallux valgus (bunion)

Alternatives

Wraps and braces can be used instead or with taping to stabilize the affected area. Braces might alter muscular activity, where tape might not.

Types of Tape

Standard Athletic Tape is classified by the following characteristics:

- Number of vertical (warp) and horizontal (woof) threads per square inch. These threads vary from 120 to 150 per square inch. A higher thread count is synonymous with a higher quality including higher tensile strength, better adhesive, easier removal, longer lasting, and more expensive.
- Tensile strength
- Composition: bleached versus unbleached cotton; cotton versus synthetic fibers versus a blend of both.
- Rigid Tape- Provides a firm support, holds and reduces movement of a joint with a strong and sticky material, examples include Strappal or Endura Fix, etc.
- Under Tape- Has a different type of fabric that allows more movement and air, examples include Hyperfix or Endura Fix, etc.
- Elastic Tape- Flexible tape when is applied that lets your skin breath and transmit moisture through the type of material used, examples include Tensoplast and Elastikon, etc.
- Felt Tape- This type of tape does not have any glue in the material and is used a barrier to the skin Example: Mueller
- Bandages- Does not have glue in the material which allows them to stick to each other Example: Coban
- Kinesio- Adjusts to skin and glides as you move, commonly used by athletes

Materials Commonly Used

- Dry Adhesive Spray
- Scissors
- Utility Emergency Shears
- Tape Remover
- Under Wrap

- Heel and Lace Pads
- Athletic Tape

Elastic Therapeutic Tape

Elastic therapeutic tape is an elastic cotton strip with an acrylic adhesive that is used with the intent of treating pain and disability from athletic injuries and a variety of other physical disorders. In individuals with chronic musculoskeletal pain, research suggests that elastic taping may help relieve pain, but not more than other treatment approaches, and there is no evidence that it can reduce disability in chronic pain cases.

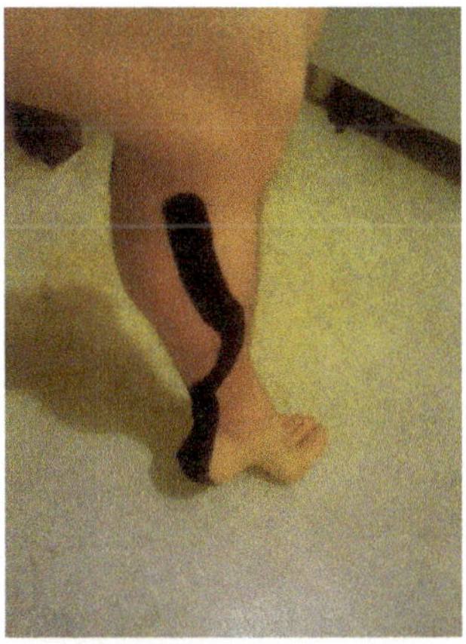

Elastic therapeutic tape applied to patient's leg

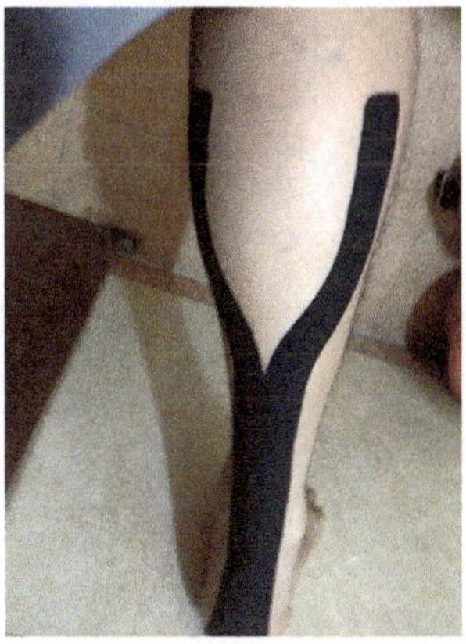

Kinesio Taping for Soleus and Achilles tendon

Properties

The product is a type of thin, elastic cotton tape that can stretch up to 140% of its original length. As a result, if the tape is applied stretched greater than its normal length, it will "recoil" after being applied and therefore create a pulling force on the skin. This elastic property allows much greater range of motion compared to traditional white athletic tape and can also be left on for long periods of time before reapplication.

Designed to mimic human skin, with roughly the same thickness and elastic properties, the tape can be stretched 30–40% in the longitudinal direction. It is a latex free material with acrylic adhesive, which is heat activated. The cotton fibers allow for evaporation and quicker drying leading to longer wear time, up to 4 days. How the tape is claimed to affect the body is dependent on its usage throughout the body and how it is applied: the direction of pull, the shape, and the location; all play a role in its hypothetical function.

There are several theoretical benefits claimed for the tape. One of those is correcting the alignment of weak muscles as well as facilitating joint motion as a result of the tape's recoiling qualities. Additionally, the tape is claimed to lift the skin, increasing the space below it, and increasing blood flow and circulation of lymphatic fluids (swelling). This increase in the interstitial space is said to lead to less pressure on the body's nociceptors, which detect pain, and to stimulate mechanoreceptors, to improve overall joint proprioception.

Effectiveness

A 2015 meta analysis found that the taping provided significantly more pain relief than no treatment at all, but was not better than other treatment approaches in patients with chronic musculoskeletal pain. The same meta analysis did not find any significant changes in disability as a result of taping. A 2012 journal article from the *Journal of Hand Therapy* suggests that kinesio tape (KT) might have some effect on lymph drainage. Based on a double blind study, KT may be of some assistance to clinicians in improving pain-free active range of motion immediately after tape application for patients with shoulder pain. Utilization of KT for decreasing pain intensity or disability for young patients with suspected shoulder tendonitis/impingement is not supported. Based on two different studies, kinesio tape showed quicker drainage than manually and better patient compliance. A 2014 meta analysis looked at methodological quality of studies along with overall population effect and suggested that studies deemed of lower methodological quality are more likely to report beneficial effects of elastic therapeutic taping. It also suggested that applying elastic therapeutic tape, "to facilitate muscular contraction has no or only negligible effects on muscle strength". A 2012 meta analysis found that the efficacy of elastic therapeutic tape in pain relief was trivial given that no studies found clinically important results. The tape "may have a small beneficial role in improving strength, range of motion in certain injured cohorts and force sense error compared with other elastic tapes, but further studies are needed to confirm these findings". The same article concluded: "KT had some substantial effects on muscle activity, but it was unclear whether these changes were beneficial or harmful. In conclusion, there was little quality evidence to support the use of KT over other types of elastic taping in the management or prevention of sports injuries."

Some researchers claim that what athletes are experiencing is a placebo effect.

Application

The tape is applied with the affected muscle in a stretched position, taping from the origin of the muscle to the insertion point. Once applied, it is rubbed to activate the pressure-sensitive adhesive.

Application is in three general shapes or techniques. An "I" shape is used for small or linear places, for example an I-shaped piece of tape will be applied to the teres minor or rhomboid minor. A "Y" shape is used for larger muscles, like the deltoid. The "X" shape is used for large and long muscles, such as the biceps femoris.

History

A surge in popularity resulted after the product was donated to Olympic athletes in the 2008 Beijing Summer Olympics and 2012 Summer Olympics.

Sports Chiropractic

Sports chiropractic is a specialty of chiropractic. It generally requires post-graduate coursework and a certification or diplomate status granted by a credentialing agency recognized in a practitioner's region. Assessment and diagnosis of sports-related injuries by a sports chiropractor involves a physical exam and sometimes imaging studies. Treatment is described as noninvasive and can include joint manipulations as well as recommendations for exercises designed to improve strength, flexibility and range of motion.

Training and Credentialing

In Canada, a two-year post-graduate program and certification as a chiropractic sports specialist (CCSS) are offered by the Royal College of Chiropractic Sports Sciences. The U.S. equivalent is the Certified Chiropractic Sports Physician (CCSP), or the Diplomate of the American Chiropractic Board of Sports Physicians (DACBSP), a three-year post-doctoral program.

The International Federation of Sports Chiropractic (FICS) established the Internationally Certified Chiropractic Sports Practitioner (ICSSP) program in connection with Murdoch University, in Perth, Australia. Applicants can receive a certification through participation in a combination of online courses and seminars, and can receive credit for post-doctoral education programs. FICS coordinates with athletic associations to provide chiropractors for international sporting events.

Use by Amateur and Professional Athletes

As of the 2014-2015 season, every NFL team had an official team chiropractor. In Major

League Baseball, 30 teams have a team chiropractor. In 2006, a study analyzing Division I NCAA athletes at intercollegiate sporting events in Hawaii found that chiropractic usage within the last 12 months was reported by 39% of respondents.

Chiropractic sports medicine specialists first began treating Olympic athletes at the Olympic Games in Montreal in 1976, when Leroy Perry began working with the Aruban team. The first official appointment of a chiropractor to the US team was during the 1980 Winter Olympic Games in Lake Placid, New York when Stephen J. Press recommended George Goodheart to the chairman of the US Olympic Committee (USOC)'s Division of Sports Medicine. Subsequently, a program was developed to screen chiropractors for the USOTC in Colorado Springs, CO and chiropractors have been included with the US and other national teams since then. In 2000, Life University opened a 4500 sq. ft. chiropractic clinic in the Costa Rican Olympic Committee Compound to provide chiropractic services for athletes. The US team sent four chiropractors to Beijing for the 2008 Olympic games, where Mike Reed served the U.S. team as a treating chiropractor and also as the chiropractic medical director of the Performance Services Division of the USOC. Chiropractors were included on the US medical team again for the 2010 Vancouver Olympic Games, where Michael Reed acted as the external medical director for the USOC, and oversaw the USOC volunteer medical program and the USOC Sports Medicine Network. Chiropractic care was arranged by the British Chiropractic Association and integrated into the treatment of athletes for a polyclinic during the 2010 Winter Olympics in Vancouver. At the 2012 Summer Games in London, the USOC brought eight chiropractors in addition to the full-time paid medical director, William Moreau.

Associations

- International Federation of Sports Chiropractic or Fédération Internationale de Chiropratique du Sport (FICS)
- International Association of Olympic Chiropractic Officers
- Royal College of Chiropractic Sport Sciences of Canada - RCCSS(C)

Physical Therapy

Physical therapy (PT), also known as physiotherapy, is a physical medicine and rehabilitation specialty that, by using mechanical force and movements, remediates impairments and promotes mobility, function, and quality of life through examination, diagnosis, prognosis, and physical intervention. It is performed by physical therapists (known as physiotherapists in many countries).

In addition to clinical practice, other activities encompassed in the physical therapy profession include research, education, consultation, and administration. Physical therapy services may be provided alongside, or in conjunction with, other medical services.

Overview

Physical therapy attempts to address the illnesses, or injuries that limit a person's abilities to move and perform functional activities in their daily lives. PTs use an individual's history and physical examination to arrive at a diagnosis and establish a management plan and, when necessary, incorporate the results of laboratory and imaging studies like X-rays, CT-scan, or MRI findings. Electrodiagnostic testing (e.g., electromyograms and nerve conduction velocity testing) may also be used. PT management commonly includes prescription of or assistance with specific exercises, manual therapy and manipulation, mechanical devices such as traction, education, physical agents which includes heat, cold, electricity, sound waves, radiation, assistive devices, prostheses, orthoses and other interventions. In addition, PTs work with individuals to prevent the loss of mobility before it occurs by developing fitness and wellness-oriented programs for healthier and more active lifestyles, providing services to individuals and populations to develop, maintain and restore maximum movement and functional ability throughout the lifespan. This includes providing therapeutic treatment in circumstances where movement and function are threatened by aging, injury, disease or environmental factors. Functional movement is central to what it means to be healthy.

Physical therapy is a professional career which has many specialties including musculoskeletal, sports, neurology, wound care, EMG, cardiopulmonary, geriatrics, orthopedics, women's health, and pediatrics. Neurological rehabilitation is in particular a rapidly emerging field. PTs practice in many settings, such as private-owned physical therapy clinics, outpatient clinics or offices, health and wellness clinics, rehabilitation hospitals facilities, skilled nursing facilities, extended care facilities, private homes, education and research centers, schools, hospices, industrial and this workplaces or other occupational environments, fitness centers and sports training facilities.

Physical therapists also practise in the non-patient care roles such as health policy, health insurance, health care administration and as health care executives. Physical therapists are involved in the medical-legal field serving as experts, performing peer review and independent medical examinations.

Education varies greatly by country. The span of education ranges from some countries having little formal education to others having doctoral degrees and post doctoral residencies and fellowships.

History

Exercise to shoulder and elbow to increase motion following fracture and dislocation of humerus is being given by an Army therapist to a soldier patient.

Physicians like Hippocrates and later Galen are believed to have been the first practitioners of physical therapy, advocating massage, manual therapy techniques and hydrotherapy to treat people in 460 BC. After the development of orthopedics in the eighteenth century, machines like the Gymnasticon were developed to treat gout and similar diseases by systematic exercise of the joints, similar to later developments in physical therapy.

The earliest documented origins of actual physical therapy as a professional group date back to Per Henrik Ling, "Father of Swedish Gymnastics," who founded the Royal Central Institute of Gymnastics (RCIG) in 1813 for manipulation, and exercise. The Swedish word for physical therapist is *sjukgymnast* = someone involved in gymnastics for those who are ill. In 1887, PTs were given official registration by Sweden's National Board of Health and Welfare. Other countries soon followed. In 1894, four nurses in Great Britain formed the Chartered Society of Physiotherapy. The School of Physiotherapy at the University of Otago in New Zealand in 1913, and the United States' 1914 Reed College in Portland, Oregon, which graduated "reconstruction aides." Since the profession's inception, spinal manipulative therapy has been a component of the physical therapist practice.

Modern physical therapy was established towards the end of the 19th century due to events that had an effect on a global scale, which called for rapid advances in physical therapy. Soon following American orthopedic surgeons began treating children with disabilities and began employing women trained in physical education, and remedial exercise. These treatments were applied and promoted further during the Polio outbreak of 1916. During the First World War women were recruited to work with and restore physical function to injured soldiers, and the field of physical therapy was institutionalized. In 1918 the term "Reconstruction Aide" was used to refer to individuals practicing physical therapy. The first school of physical therapy was established at Walter Reed Army Hospital in Washington, D.C., following the outbreak of World War I. Research catalyzed the physical therapy movement. The first physical therapy research was published in the United States in March 1921 in "The PT Review." In the same year, Mary McMillan organized the American Women's Physical Therapeutic Association (now called the American Physical Therapy Association (APTA). In 1924, the Georgia Warm Springs Foundation promoted the field by touting physical therapy as a treatment for polio. Treatment through the 1940s primarily consisted of exercise, massage, and traction. Manipulative procedures to the spine and extremity joints began to be practiced, especially in the British Commonwealth countries, in the early 1950s. Around this time when polio vaccines were developed, physical therapists have become a normal occurrence in hospitals throughout North America and Europe. In the late 1950s, physical therapists started to move beyond hospital-based practice to outpatient orthopedic clinics, public schools, colleges/universities health-centres, geriatric settings (skilled nursing facilities), rehabilitation centers and medical centers. Specialization for physical therapy in the U.S. occurred in 1974, with the Orthopaedic Section of the APTA being formed for those physical therapists specializing in orthopaedics. In the same year, the International Federation of Orthopaedic Manipulative Physical Therapists was formed, which has ever since played an important role in advancing manual therapy worldwide.

Education

Educational criteria for physical therapy providers vary from state to state and from country to country, and among various levels of professional responsibility. Most U.S. states have physical therapy practice acts that recognize both physical therapists (PT) and physical therapist assistants (PTA) and some jurisdictions also recognize physical therapy technicians (PT Techs) or aides. Most countries have licensing bodies that require physical therapists to be a member of before they can start practicing as independent professionals.

Canada

Canadian Physiotherapy programs are offered at 15 Universities, often through the university's respective college of medicine. In the past decade, each of Canada's physical therapy schools has transitioned from 3-year Bachelor of Science in Physical Therapy (BScPT) programs that required 2 years of pre-requisites university courses (5-year bachelor's degree) to 2-year Master's of Physical Therapy (MPT) programs that require pre-requisite bachelor's degrees. The last Canadian university to follow suit was the University of Manitoba who transitioned to the MPT program in 2012, making the MPT credential the new entry to practice standard across Canada. Existing practitioners with BScPT credentials are not required to upgrade their qualifications.

In the province of Quebec, prospective physiotherapists are required to have completed a college diploma in either health sciences, which lasts on average two years, or physical rehabilitation technology, which lasts at least three years, to apply to a physiotherapy program or program in university. Following admission, physical therapy students work on a bachelor of science with a major in physical therapy and rehabilitation. The B.Sc. usually requires three years to complete. Students must then enter graduate school to complete a master's degree in physical therapy, which normally requires one and a half to two years of study. Graduates who obtain their M.Sc. must successfully pass the membership examination to become member of the Ordre professionnel de la physiothérapie du Québec (OPPQ). Physiotherapists can pursue their education in such fields as rehabilitation sciences, sports medicine, kinesiology, and physiology.

In the province of Quebec, physical rehabilitation therapists are health care professionals who are required to complete a three-year college diploma program in physical rehabilitation therapy and be member of the *Ordre professionnel de la physiothérapie du Québec* (OPPQ) in order to practise legally in the country.

Most physical rehabilitation therapists complete their college diploma at Collège Montmorency, Dawson College, or Cégep Marie-Victorin, all situated in and around the Montreal area.

After completing their technical college diploma, graduates have the opportunity to pursue their studies at the university level to perhaps obtain a bachelor's degree in physiotherapy, kinesiology, exercise science, or occupational therapy. The Université de Montréal, the Université Laval and the Université de Sherbrooke are among the Québécois universities that admit physical rehabilitation therapists in their programs of study related to health sciences and rehabilitation in order to credit courses that were completed in college.

To date, there are no bridging programs available to facilitate upgrading from the BScPT to the MPT credential. However, research Master's of Science (MSc) and Doctor of Philosophy (PhD) programs are available at every university. Aside from academic research, practitioners can upgrade their skills and qualifications through continuing education courses and curriculums. Continuing education is a requirement of the provincial regulatory bodies.

The Canadian Alliance of Physiotherapy Regulators (CAPR), or simply known as The Alliance, offers eligible program graduates to apply for the national Physiotherapy Competency Examination (PCE). Passing the PCE is one of the requirements in most provinces and territories to work as a licensed physiotherapist in Canada. The Alliance has members which are physiotherapy regulatory organizations recognized in their respective provinces and territories:

- Government of Yukon, Consumer Services
- College of Physical Therapists of British Columbia
- Physiotherapy Alberta College + Association
- Saskatchewan College of Physical Therapists
- College of Physiotherapists of Manitoba
- College of Physiotherapists of Ontario
- Ordre professionnel de la physiothérapie du Québec
- College of Physiotherapists of New Brunswick/Collège des physiothérapeutes du Nouveau-Brunswick
- Nova Scotia College of Physiotherapists
- Prince Edward Island College of Physiotherapists
- Newfoundland & Labrador College of Physiotherapists

The Canadian Physiotherapy Association offers a curriculum of continuing education courses in orthopaedics and manual therapy. The program consists of 5 levels (7 courses) of training with ongoing mentorship and evaluation at each level. The orthopaedic curriculum and examinations takes a minimum of 4 years to complete. However, upon completion of level 2, physiotherapists can apply to a unique 1-year course-based Master's program in advanced orthopaedics and manipulation at the University of Western Ontario to complete their training. This program accepts only 16 physiotherapists annually since 2007. Successful completion of either of these education streams and their respective examinations allows physiotherapists the opportunity to apply to the Canadian Academy of Manipulative Physiotherapy (CAMPT) for fellowship. Fellows of the Canadian Academy of manipulative Physiotherapists (FCAMPT) are considered leaders in the field, having extensive post-graduate education in orthopaedics and manual therapy. FCAMPT is an internationally recognized credential, as CAMPT is a member of the International Federation of Manipulative Physiotherapists (IFOMPT), a branch of the World Confederation of Physical Therapy (WCPT) and the World Health Organization (WHO).

Scotland

Physiotherapy degrees are offered at three universities: Robert Gordon University in Aberdeen, Glasgow Caledonian University in Glasgow and Queen Margaret University in Edinburgh. Students can qualify as physiotherapists by completing a four-year Bachelor of Science degree or a two-year master's degree (if they already have an undergraduate degree in a related field).

In order to use the title 'Physiotherapist', a student must register with the Health and Care Professions Council, a UK wide regulatory body, on qualifying. Many physiotherapists are also members of the Chartered Society of Physiotherapists (CSP), who provides insurance and professional support.

United States

The primary physical therapy practitioner is the Physical Therapist (PT) who is trained and licensed to examine, evaluate, diagnose and treat impairment, functional limitations and disabilities in patients or clients. Physical therapist education curricula in the United States culminate in a Doctor of Physical Therapy (DPT) degree, but many currently practising PTs hold a Master of Physical Therapy degree, and some still hold a Bachelor's degree. Currently the education programs for physical therapy have changed. The Master of Physical Therapy and Master of Science in Physical Therapy degrees are no longer offered, and the entry-level degree is the Doctor of Physical Therapy degree, which typically takes 3 years. PTs who hold a Masters or bachelors in PT are encouraged to get their DPT because APTA's goal is for all PT's to be on a doctoral level. WCPT recommends physical therapist entry-level educational programs be based on university or university-level studies, of a minimum of four years, independently validated and accredited. Curricula in the United States are accredited by the Commission on Accreditation in Physical Therapy Education (CAPTE). According to CAPTE, as of 2017 there are 31,380 students currently enrolled in 227 accredited PT programs in the

United States while 12,945 PTA students are currently enrolled in 331 PTA programs in the United States. Updated CAPTE statistics list that for 2015-2016, there are 30,419 students enrolled in 233 accredited PT programs in the United States.

The physical therapist professional curriculum includes content in the clinical sciences (e.g., content about the cardiovascular, pulmonary, endocrine, metabolic, gastrointestinal, genitourinary, integumentary, musculoskeletal, and neuromuscular systems and the medical and surgical conditions frequently seen by physical therapists). Current training is specifically aimed to enable physical therapists to appropriately recognize and refer non-musculoskeletal diagnoses that may presently similarly to those caused by systems not appropriate for physical therapy intervention, which has resulted in direct access to physical therapists in many states.

Post-doctoral residency and fellowship education prevalence is increasing steadily with 219 residency, and 42 fellowship programs accredited in 2016. Residencies are aimed to train physical therapists in a specialty such as acute care, cardiovascular & pulmonary, clinical electrophysiology, faculty, geriatrics, neurology, orthopaedics, pediatrics, sports, women's health, and wound care, whereas fellowships train specialists in a subspecialty (e.g. critical care, hand therapy, and division 1 sports), similar to the medical model. Residency programs offer eligibility to sit for the specialist certification in their respective area of practice. For example, completion of an orthopaedic physical therapy residency, allows its graduates to apply and sit for the clinical specialist examination in orthopaedics, achieving the OCS designation upon passing the examination. Board certification of physical therapy specialists is aimed to recognize individuals with advanced clinical knowledge and skill training in their respective area of practice, and exemplifies the trend toward greater education to optimally treat individuals with movement dysfunction.

Physical therapist assistants may deliver treatment and physical interventions for patients and clients under a care plan established by and under the supervision of a physical therapist. Physical therapist assistants in the United States are currently trained under associate of applied sciences curricula specific to the profession, as outlined and accredited by CAPTE. As of August 2011, there were 276 accredited two-year (Associate degree) programs for physical therapist assistants In the United States of America. According to CAPTE, as of 2012 there are 10,598 students currently enrolled in 280 accredited PTA programs in the United States. Updated CAPTE statistics list that for 2015-2016, there are 12,726 students enrolled in 340 accredited PTA programs in the United States.

Curricula for the physical therapist assistant associate degree include:

- Anatomy & physiology
- Exercise physiology
- Human biology

- Physics
- Biomechanics
- Kinesiology
- Neuroscience
- Clinical pathology
- Behavioral sciences
- Communication
- Ethics
- Research
- Other coursework as required by individual programs.

Job duties and education requirements for Physical Therapy Technicians or Aides may vary depending on the employer, but education requirements range from high school diploma or equivalent to completion of a 2-year degree program. O-Net reports that 64% of PT Aides/Techs have a high school diploma or equivalent, 21% have completed some college but do not hold a degree, and 10% hold an associate degree.

Some jurisdictions allow physical therapists to employ technicians or aides or therapy assistants to perform designated routine tasks related to physical therapy under the direct supervision of a physical therapist. Some jurisdictions require physical therapy technicians or aides to be certified, and education and certification requirements vary among jurisdictions.

Employment

Physical therapy-related jobs in North America have shown rapid growth in recent years, but employment rates and average wages may vary significantly between different countries, states, provinces or regions. A study from 2013 states that 56.4% of physical therapists were globally satisfied with their jobs. Salary, interest in work, and fulfillment in job are important predictors of job satisfaction. In a Polish study, job burnout among the physical therapists was manifested by increased emotional exhaustion and decreased sense of personal achievement. Emotional exhaustion is significantly higher among physical therapists working with adults and employed in hospitals. Other factors that increased burnout include working in a hospital setting and having seniority from 15 to 19 years.

United States of America

According to the United States Department of Labor's Bureau of Labor Statistics, there were approximately 210,900 physical therapists employed in the United States in 2014, earning an average $84,020 annually in 2015, or $40.40 per hour, with 34% growth in employment projected by the year 2024. The Bureau of Labor Statistics also reports that there were approximately 128,700 Physical Therapist Assistants and Aides employed in the United States in 2014, earning an average $42,980 annually, or $20.66 per hour, with 40% growth in employment projected by the year 2024. To meet their needs, many healthcare and physical therapy facilities hire "travel physical therapists", who work temporary assignments between 8 and 26 weeks for much higher wages; about $113,500 a year. Bureau of Labor Statistics data on PTAs and Techs can be difficult to decipher, due to their tendency to report data on these job fields collectively rather than separately. O-Net reports that in 2015, PTAs in the United States earned a median wage of $55,170 annually or $26.52 hourly, and that Aides/Techs earned a median wage of $25,120 annually or $12.08 hourly in 2015. The American Physical Therapy Association reports vacancy rates for physical therapists as 11.2% in outpatient private practice, 10% in acute care settings, and 12.1% in skilled nursing facilities. The APTA also reports turnover rates for physical therapists as 10.7% in outpatient private practice, 11.9% in acute care settings, 27.6% in skilled nursing facilities.

Specialty Areas

The body of knowledge of physical therapy is large, and therefore physical therapists may specialize in a specific clinical area. While there are many different types of physical therapy, the American Board of Physical Therapy Specialties lists nine current specialist certifications, the ninth, Oncology, pending for its first examination in 2019. Most Physical Therapists practicing in a specialty will have undergone further training, such as an accredited residency program, although individuals are currently able to sit for their specialist examination after 2,000 hours of focused practice in their respective specialty population, in addition to requirements set by each respective specialty board.

Cardiovascular and Pulmonary Physiotherapy

Cardiovascular and pulmonary rehabilitation respiratory practitioners and physical therapists offer therapy for a wide variety of cardiopulmonary disorders or pre and post cardiac or pulmonary surgery. An example of cardiac surgery is coronary bypass surgery. Primary goals of this specialty include increasing endurance and functional independence. Manual therapy is used in this field to assist in clearing lung secretions experienced with cystic fibrosis. Pulmonary disorders, heart attacks, post coronary bypass surgery, chronic obstructive pulmonary disease, and pulmonary fibrosis, treatments can benefit from cardiovascular and pulmonary specialized physical therapists.

Clinical Electrophysiology

This specialty area includes electrotherapy/physical agents, electrophysiological evaluation (EMG/NCV), physical agents, and wound management.

Geriatric

Geriatric physical therapy covers a wide area of issues concerning people as they go through normal adult aging but is usually focused on the older adult. There are many conditions that affect many people as they grow older and include but are not limited to the following: arthritis, osteoporosis, cancer, Alzheimer's disease, hip and joint replacement, balance disorders, incontinence, etc. Geriatric physical therapists specialize in providing therapy for such conditions in older adults.

Integumentary

Integumentary physical therapy includes the treatment of conditions involving the skin and all its related organs. Common conditions managed include wounds and burns. Physical therapists may utilize surgical instruments, wound irrigations, dressings and topical agents to remove the damaged or contaminated tissue and promote tissue healing. Other commonly used interventions include exercise, edema control, splinting, and compression garments. The work done by physical therapists in the integumentary specialty do work similar to what would be done by medical doctors or nurses in the emergency room or triage.

Neurological

Neurological physical therapy is a field focused on working with individuals who have a neurological disorder or disease. These can include stroke, chronic back pain, Alzheimer's disease, Charcot-Marie-Tooth disease (CMT), ALS, brain injury, cerebral palsy, l.g.b. syndrome, multiple sclerosis, Parkinson's disease, facial palsy and spinal cord injury. Common impairments associated with neurologic conditions include impairments of vision, balance, ambulation, activities of daily living, movement, muscle strength and loss of functional independence. The techniques involve in neurological physical therapy are wide-ranging and often require specialized training.

Neurological physiotherapy is also called neurophysiotherapy or neurological rehabilitation.

Orthopedic

Orthopedic physical therapists diagnose, manage, and treat disorders and injuries of the musculoskeletal system including rehabilitation after orthopedic surgery. acute trauma such as sprains, strains,injuries of insidious onset such as tendinopathy, bursitis and deformities like scoliosis. This speciality of physical therapy is most often found in the out-patient clinical setting. Orthopedic therapists are trained in the treatment of post-operative orthopedic procedures, fractures, acute sports injuries, arthritis, sprains, strains, back and neck pain, spinal conditions, and amputations.

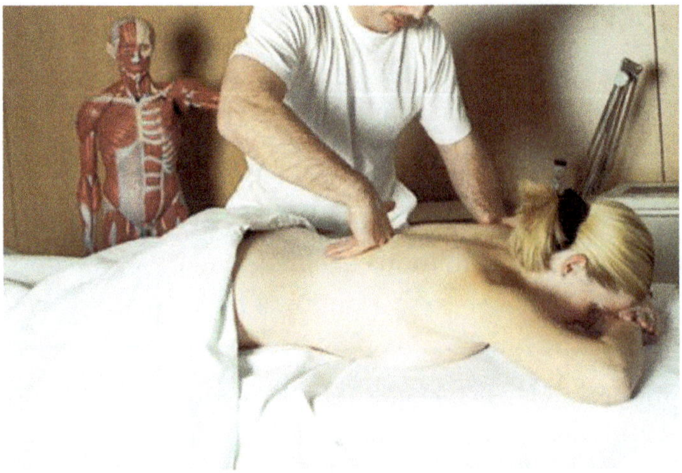

Treatment by orthopedic physical therapists

Joint and spine mobilization/manipulation, dry needling (similar to acupuncture), therapeutic exercise, neuromuscular techniques, muscle reeducation, hot/cold packs, and electrical muscle stimulation (e.g., cryotherapy, iontophoresis, electrotherapy) are modalities employed to expedite recovery in the orthopedic setting. Additionally, an emerging adjunct to diagnosis and treatment is the use of sonography for diagnosis and to guide treatments such as muscle retraining. Those who have suffered injury or disease affecting the muscles, bones, ligaments, or tendons will benefit from assessment by a physical therapist specialized in orthopedics.

Pediatric

Pediatric physical therapy assists in early detection of health problems and uses a variety of modalities to provide physical therapy for disorders in the pediatric population. These therapists are specialized in the diagnosis, treatment, and management of infants, children, and adolescents with a variety of congenital, developmental, neuromuscular, skeletal, or acquired disorders/diseases. Treatments focus mainly on improving gross and fine motor skills, balance and coordination, strength and endurance as well as cognitive and sensory processing/integration.

Sports

Physical therapists are closely involved in the care and wellbeing of athletes including recreational, semi-professional (paid) and professional (full-time employment) participants. This area of practice encompasses athletic injury management under 5 main categories:

1. acute care – assessment and diagnosis of an initial injury;
2. treatment – application of specialist advice and techniques to encourage healing;

3. rehabilitation – progressive management for full return to sport;
4. prevention – identification and address of deficiencies known to directly result in, or act as precursors to injury, such as movement assessment
5. education – sharing of specialist knowledge to individual athletes, teams or clubs to assist in prevention or management of injury

Physical therapists who work for professional sport teams often have a specialized sports certification issued through their national registering organisation. Most Physical therapists who practice in a sporting environment are also active in collaborative sports medicine programs too.

Women's Health

Women's health physical therapy mostly addresses women's issues related to the female reproductive system, child birth, and post-partum. These conditions include lymphedema, osteoporosis, pelvic pain, prenatal and post-partum periods, and urinary incontinence. It also addresses incontinence, pelvic pain, and other disorders associated with pelvic floor dysfunction. Manual physical therapy has been demonstrated in multiple studies to increase rates of conception in women with infertility.

Palliative Care

Physiotherapy in the field of oncology and palliative care is a continuously evolving and developing specialty, both in malignant and non-malignant diseases. Rehabilitation for both groups of patients is now recognized as an essential part of the clinical pathway, as early diagnoses and new treatments are enabling patients to live longer. it is generally accepted that patients should have access to an appropriate level of rehabilitation, so that they can function at a minimum level of dependency and optimize their quality of life, regardless of their life expectancy.

Back Pain Treatment

Physiotherapy is scientifically proven to be one of the most effective ways to treat and prevent pain and injury.It strengthens muscles and improves function.

It not only reduces or removes pain for a short time, but also reduces the risk for future back-pain re-occurrence. Based on the particular diagnosis, varied methods are practiced by physiotherapists to treat patients. They may follow pain management program, which helps get rid of inflammation and swelling for sometimes.

Physical Therapist–patient Collaborative Relationship

A systematic review that included patients with brain injury, musculoskeletal conditions, cardiac conditions, or multiple pathologies found that the alliance between patient and therapist positively correlates with treatment outcome. Outcomes includes: ability to perform activities of daily living, manage pain, complete specific physical function tasks, depression, global assessment of physical health, treatment adherence, and treatment satisfaction.

Studies have explored four themes that may influence patient–therapist interactions: interpersonal and communication skills, practical skills, individualized patient-centered care, and organizational and environmental factors. Physical therapists need to be able to effectively communicate with their patients on a variety of levels. Patients have varying levels of health literacy so it is important for physical therapists to take that into account when discussing the patient's ailments as well as planned treatment. Research has shown that using communication tools tailored to the patient's health literacy leads to improved engagement with their practitioner and their clinical care. In addition, patients reported that shared decision-making will yield a positive relationship. Practical skills such as the ability to educate patients about their conditions, and professional expertise are perceived as valuable factors in patient care. Patients value the ability of a clinician to provide clear and simple explanations about their problems. Furthermore, patients value when physical therapists possess excellent technical skills that improve the patient effectively.

Environmental factors such as the location, equipment used, and parking are less important to the patient than the physical therapy clinical encounter itself.

Based on the current understanding, the most important factors that contribute to the patient–therapist interactions include that the physical therapist: spends an adequate amount of time with the patient, possesses strong listening and communication skills, treats the patient with respect, provides clear explanations of the treatment, and allows the patient to be involved in the treatment decisions.

Effectiveness

A 2012 systematic review found evidence to support the use of spine manipulation by physical therapists as a safe option to improve outcomes for low back pain. A 2015 systematic review suggested that spine manipulation and therapeutic massage are effective interventions for neck pain; it also suggested, however, that electroacupuncture, strain-counterstrain, relaxation massage, heat therapy and ultrasound therapy are not effective and thus not recommended for the treatment of neck pain.

Telehealth

Telehealth (or telerehabilitation) is a developing form of physical therapy to respond to the increasing demand and high cost of typical physical therapy treatment. Telehealth is online communication between the clinician and patient either live or in prerecorded sessions.The benefits of telehealth include improved accessibility in remote areas, more cost efficient services, improved convenience for the home-bound and physically disabled. Some considerations for telehealth are limited evidence to prove effectiveness and compliance more than in-person therapy, licensure and payment policy issues, compromised privacy. Studies are controversial as to the effectiveness of telehealth in patients with various conditions, such as stroke, multiple sclerosis and lower back pain.

United States

Definitions and licensing requirements in the United States vary among jurisdictions, as each state has enacted its own physical therapy practice act defining the profession within its jurisdiction, but the American Physical Therapy Association (APTA) has also drafted a model definition in order to limit this variation, and the APTA is also responsible for accrediting physical therapy education curricula throughout the United States of America.

Ulnar Collateral Ligament Reconstruction

Ulnar collateral ligament reconstruction, also known as Tommy John surgery (TJS), is a surgical graft procedure in which the ulnar collateral ligament in the medial elbow is replaced with either a tendon from elsewhere from the patient's own body, or the use of a tendon from the donated tissue of a cadaver. The procedure is common among collegiate and professional athletes in several sports, most notably baseball.

The procedure was first performed in 1974 by orthopedic surgeon Frank Jobe, then a Los Angeles Dodgers team physician who served as a special advisor to the team until his death in 2014. It is named after the first baseball player to undergo the surgery, major league pitcher Tommy John, whose record of 288 career victories ranks seventh all time among left-handed pitchers. The initial operation, John's successful post-surgery career, and the relationship between the two men is the subject of a 2013 ESPN *30 for 30* documentary.

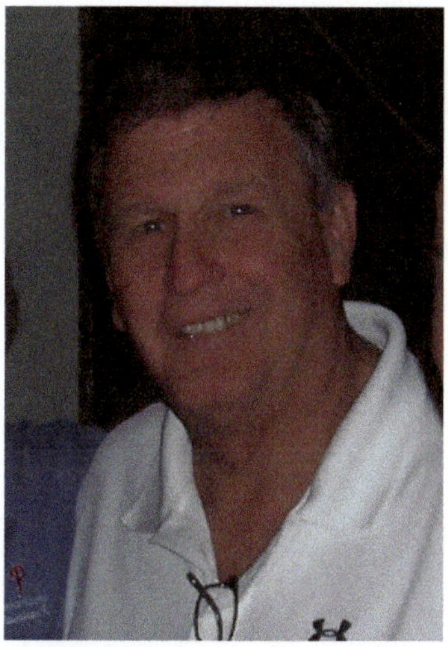

Tommy John, for whom the surgery is named, in 2008

At the time of Tommy John's operation, Dr. Jobe put the chances for success of the operation at 1 in 100. In 2009, prospects of a complete recovery had risen to 85–92 percent.

Following his 1974 surgery, John missed the entire 1975 season rehabilitating his arm before returning for the 1976 season. Before his surgery, John had won 124 games. He won 164 games after surgery, retiring in 1989 at age 46.

For baseball players, full rehabilitation takes about one year for pitchers and about six months for position players. Players typically begin throwing about 16 weeks after surgery. While eighty percent of players return to pitching at the same level as before the surgery, for those Major League pitchers who receive the surgery twice, thirty five percent do not return to pitch in the majors at all.

Injury Factors

The ulnar collateral ligament (UCL) can become stretched, frayed, or torn through the repetitive stress of the throwing motion. The risk of injury to the throwing athlete's UCL is thought to be extremely high as the amount of stress through this structure approaches its ultimate tensile strength during a hard throw.

While many authorities suggest that an individual's style of throwing or the type of pitches they throw are the most important determinant of their likelihood to sustain an injury, the results of a 2002 study suggest that the total number of pitches thrown is the greatest determinant. A 2002 study examined the throwing volume, pitch type, and throwing mechanics of 426 pitchers aged 9 to 14 for one year. Compared to pitchers who threw 200 or fewer pitches in a season, those who threw 201–400, 401–600, 601–800, and 800+ pitches faced an increased risk of 63%, 181%, 234%, and 161% respectively. The types of pitches thrown showed a smaller effect; throwing a slider was associated with an 86% increased chance of elbow injury, while throwing a curveball was associated with an increase in pain. There was only a weak correlation between throwing mechanics perceived as bad and injury-prone. Thus, although there is a large body of other evidence that suggests mistakes in throwing mechanics increase the likelihood of injury it seems that the greater risk lies in the volume of throwing in total. Research into the area of throwing injuries in young athletes has led to age-based recommendations for pitch limits for young athletes. A 2016 study explained 22% of the variation in those needing ulnar collateral ligament reconstruction, citing handedness, standard deviation of release point, days lost to arm and shoulder injuries, previous ulnar collateral ligament reconstruction, number of hard pitches, ERA-, and age as the known risk factors.

In younger athletes, whose epiphyseal plate (growth plate) is still open, the force on the inside of the elbow during throwing is more likely to cause the elbow to fail at this point than at the ulnar collateral ligament. This injury is often termed "Little League elbow" and can be serious but does not require reconstructing the UCL.

Increasingly often, pitchers require a second procedure after returning to pitching –

the periods from 2001–2012 and 2013–2015 both saw eighteen Major League pitchers receiving the procedure a second time. As of April 2015, the average amount of time between procedures is 4.97 years.

Surgical Procedure

A 3–4 inch surgical incision is made near the elbow. Holes to accommodate a replacement graft tendon are drilled in the ulna and humerus bones of the elbow. A harvested tendon, such as the palmaris tendon from the forearm of the same or opposite elbow, the patellar tendon, hamstring, toe extensor or a donor tendon (allograft), is then woven in a figure-eight pattern through the holes and anchored. The ulnar nerve is usually moved to prevent pain as scar tissue can apply pressure to the nerve. The procedure is done on an outpatient basis allowing a return to home the same day, with the arm in a splint to protect the repair for the first week. After one week, a brace is employed to protect the reconstruction for about 6 weeks following surgery.

Risk

There is a risk of damage to the ulnar nerve.

Misconceptions

Some baseball pitchers believe they can throw harder after ulnar collateral ligament reconstruction than they did beforehand. As a result, orthopedic surgeons have reported that parents of young pitchers have come to them and asked them to perform the procedure on their un-injured sons in the hope that this will increase their sons' performance. However, many people—including Dr. Frank Jobe—believe any post-surgical increases in performance are most likely due to the increased stability of the elbow joint and pitchers' increased attention to their fitness and conditioning. Jobe believed that, rather than allowing pitchers to gain speed, the surgery and rehab protocols merely allow pitchers to return to their pre-injury levels of performance.

Adolescence

Over the last two decades, the number of UCLR surgeries has increased 3–fold, an incidence expected to rise in upcoming years. A study of youths who underwent UCLR surgery showed that boys and girls aged 15 to 19 had more surgical procedures than any other age group, with the rate of surgeries performed on 15 to 19 year olds increasing by 9% per year.

USA Baseball, Major League Baseball and Little League Baseball have initiated the Pitch Smart program designed to decrease risk of elbow injuries in adolescent pitchers. The main risk factors for elbow injury from overhead throwing include number of pitches per game, innings pitched per season, months pitched per year and poor pitching biomechanics which may increase torque and force on the elbow.

References

- De Conde, C. (1990). The CATA – A Historical Perspective. The Journal of the Canadian Athletic Therapists' Association, 6–10
- Press, Stephen J. (2013), History of Sports Chiropractic, New Jersey: C.I.S Commercial Finance Grp., Ltd., pp. 73–75, ISBN 9781105536830
- Kahanov, EdD, ATC, Leamor. "Kinesio Taping: An Overview of Use With Athletes, Part II". Alternative & Complementary Concepts. Retrieved 24 October 2012. CS1 maint: Multiple names: authors list (link)
- Bunce SM, Moore AP, Hough AD (May 2002). "M-mode ultrasound: a reliable measure of transversus abdominis thickness?". Clin Biomech (Bristol, Avon). 17 (4): 315–7. PMID 12034127. doi:10.1016/S0268-0033(02)00011-6
- Bandyopadhyay, Amit; Mahapatra, Dakshayani (2012). "Taping in Sports: a brief update". Journal of Human Sport and Exercise. 7 (2): 544–552. doi:10.4100/jhse.2012.72.17
- Press, DC, PhD, Stephen J. (2012). The History of Sports Chiropractic (Ass'n for the History of Chiropractic ed.). USA: C.I.S. Commercial Fin. Grp, Ltd. p. 495. ISBN 9781105536830. CS1 maint: Multiple names: authors list (link)
- "Continuing Education - Certificate for a Chiropractic Sports Physician 2009 - CCSP Program". Parker College of Chiropractic. Archived from the original on October 12, 2008. Retrieved 2008-04-19
- Fleisig, G. S.; Andrews, J. R. (2012). "Prevention of Elbow Injuries in Youth Baseball Pitchers". Sports Health: A Multidisciplinary Approach. 4 (5): 419–424. PMC 3435945. PMID 23016115. doi:10.1177/1941738112454828
- Bassett K, Lingman S, Ellis R (2010). "The use and treatment efficacy of kinaesthetic taping for musculoskeletal conditions: A systematic review". New Zealand Journal of Physiotherapy
- American Physical Therapy Association (17 January 2008). "APTA Background Sheet 2008". American Physical Therapy Association. Archived from the original on 29 May 2008. Retrieved 29 May 2008
- Purcell, Derek B; Matava, Matthew J; Wright, Rick W (2007). "Ulnar Collateral Ligament Reconstruction". Clinical Orthopaedics and Related Research. 455: 72–7. PMID 17279038. doi:10.1097/BLO.0b013e31802eb447
- af Klinteberg, Margareta (1992). "The History and Present Scope of Physical Therapy". International Journal of Technology Assessment in Health Care. 8 (1): 4–9. PMID 1601592. doi:10.1017/s0266462300007856
- McKenzie, R A (1998). The Cervical and Thoracic Spine: Mechanical Diagnosis and Therapy. New Zealand: Spinal Publications Ltd. pp. 16–20. ISBN 978-0-9597746-7-2
- Vancouver Organizing Committee. "2010 Winter Olympics Games Business Plan and Games Budget" (PDF). p. 151. Archived from the original (PDF) on August 30, 2008. Retrieved
- Kirti Sundar Sahu, Bhavna Bharati (2014). "Role of Physiotherapy in Public Health Domain: India Perspective". Indian Journal of Physiotherapy & Occupational Therapy. 8: 134–7
- Cameron, Michelle H. (2003). Physical agents in rehabilitation: from research to practice. Philadelphia: W. B. Saunders. ISBN 0-7216-9378-4

Permissions

All chapters in this book are published with permission under the Creative Commons Attribution Share Alike License or equivalent. Every chapter published in this book has been scrutinized by our experts. Their significance has been extensively debated. The topics covered herein carry significant information for a comprehensive understanding. They may even be implemented as practical applications or may be referred to as a beginning point for further studies.

We would like to thank the editorial team for lending their expertise to make the book truly unique. They have played a crucial role in the development of this book. Without their invaluable contributions this book wouldn't have been possible. They have made vital efforts to compile up to date information on the varied aspects of this subject to make this book a valuable addition to the collection of many professionals and students.

This book was conceptualized with the vision of imparting up-to-date and integrated information in this field. To ensure the same, a matchless editorial board was set up. Every individual on the board went through rigorous rounds of assessment to prove their worth. After which they invested a large part of their time researching and compiling the most relevant data for our readers.

The editorial board has been involved in producing this book since its inception. They have spent rigorous hours researching and exploring the diverse topics which have resulted in the successful publishing of this book. They have passed on their knowledge of decades through this book. To expedite this challenging task, the publisher supported the team at every step. A small team of assistant editors was also appointed to further simplify the editing procedure and attain best results for the readers.

Apart from the editorial board, the designing team has also invested a significant amount of their time in understanding the subject and creating the most relevant covers. They scrutinized every image to scout for the most suitable representation of the subject and create an appropriate cover for the book.

The publishing team has been an ardent support to the editorial, designing and production team. Their endless efforts to recruit the best for this project, has resulted in the accomplishment of this book. They are a veteran in the field of academics and their pool of knowledge is as vast as their experience in printing. Their expertise and guidance has proved useful at every step. Their uncompromising quality standards have made this book an exceptional effort. Their encouragement from time to time has been an inspiration for everyone.

The publisher and the editorial board hope that this book will prove to be a valuable piece of knowledge for students, practitioners and scholars across the globe.

Index